D0562938

Why Can't I Stay Motivated?

Eight steps to design your life for
successful, permanent weight loss

by
Lorrie Medford, C.N.

LDN Publishing
P.O. Box 54007
Tulsa, Oklahoma 74155

WHY CAN'T I STAY MOTIVATED?
Eight Steps to Design Your Life for Successful, Permanent Weight Loss
ISBN #0-9676419-2-6
Copyright © 2001 Lorrie Medford, C.N.
LDN Publishing
P. O. Box 54007
Tulsa, OK 74155

Unless otherwise indicated, all Scripture quotations are taken from the *King James Version* of the Bible.

Library of Congress Cataloging-in-Publishing Data

Medford, Lorrie, 1949

> Why Can't I Stay Motivated?
> Lorrie Medford, C.N.
> International Standard Book Number: 0-9676419-2-6
> 1. Weight loss 2. Motivation (Psychology) 3. Success I.Title

NOTE: This program is designed for healthy adults. If you have special health needs such as chronic disease, diabetes, heart conditions, pregnancy or are a lactating woman, or have a medical condition that requires medical attention, consult your health care provider for assistance and advice before beginning this program.

Printed in the United States of America

10 9 8 7 6 5 4 3 2 1 First U. S. Edition

(For ordering information, refer to the back pages of this book.)

The names of my clients have been changed. Any similarity to a real person is purely coincidental.

"What a great book! Lorrie has pulled together a simple, quick, easy-to-read book that truly delivers a comprehensive program for weight loss. As I read this book, I felt Lorrie was right across from me sharing her personal experiences and challenges as she overcame the hurdles of losing weight. This is a great inspirational book that will help many people successfully lose weight and achieve a healthier state."

Charles C. Dubois,
President, Standard Process, Inc.
West Palmyra, Wisconsin

"Wow! Lorrie Medford hits the mark with this incredible holistic approach to weight loss and behavioral change! Lorrie addresses the physical, mental-emotional and the spiritual needs of an individual in their pursuit of becoming the person that they are meant to be! She combines scientific nutritional knowledge with the science of motivation in this guide to weight management. Yes, with Why Can't I Stay Motivated, you will never need to buy another weight loss book again!"

John Irvin, C.S.P.
President, Lifestyle Enhancement Services, Inc.
Author, *Chicken Poop for Your Bowl*
Tulsa, Oklahoma

"Lorrie's book is more than a successful plan for weight control; it is a motivational tool for life. We found ourselves motivated to pursue dormant dreams and shelved projects. Wow! Meeting Lorrie changed our lives, and this book will change our future! It will change your life, too!"

"Armadillo Jim" and Sheila Schmidt
President/Founder, Put On Your Armor Foundation
Broken Arrow, Oklahoma

Dedication

This book is dedicated to my twin sister, Jackie, her husband, Robert and their precious children—Matthew, Kenath, David and Timothy Johnson. You are a godly family, and I delight in what God is doing in your lives to touch people in Egypt.

Contents

Foreword

As an author, syndicated columnist, public speaker, and host of a TV interview show, I have long been a student of human behavior. Each year for the past several decades, there is an annual survey conducted to determine what is the greatest desire for change among average people in our society. Every year, the top three answers have remained consistent. The third most popular answer is people want to be in a great relationship. The second most popular answer is people want more money. The most popular answer, year after year, is that people want to lose weight. As someone who has recently lost well over 100 pounds myself, I have fallen into that most popular category for most of my adult life.

Lorrie Medford's book is timely, easy-to-read, and packed with practical tips that she used to not only lose weight and keep it off, but to change her life. She also has clinical experience with thousands of people who have lost weight and also changed their lives in the process. Her book can be a turning point in your life.

I encourage you to not only read Lorrie's book, but to follow her step-by-step principles of change. As Lorrie says in her book, losing weight is not just a physical problem, but is also emotional, spiritual, and psychological. You will have to see yourself at your ideal weight and condition long before it will manifest itself and allow the rest of the world to see you that way. This book won't provide you with a magic pill or secret diet tip. Those magic fixes simply do not exist in the real world where you and I live. This book will help you to begin making changes that will not only result in weight loss, but a new attitude, which will affect your finances, relationships, and every area of your personal and professional life.

I look forward to your success.

Jim Stovall
President
Narrative Television Network
Emmy Award Winner
Gold Medalist Olympian

Acknowledgements

So many people have encouraged me to write this book, and I am grateful to every one of them. I am most grateful to my clients, and pray that this book will help them to move further in their goals for a healthy lifestyle. Thank you, especially to Anne Spears and Carolyn Clark, my two wonderful assistants who are so willing to serve my clients with a pure heart. Anne helped me name this book when she asked me one day, "Why can't I stay motivated?" Thanks for all you do for me, and for helping me to put this book together to answer that very question!

Many people read my manuscript at various stages. I am most grateful to my friend, Jim Stovall for writing my foreword, but also for encouraging me as a writer and speaker, along with other Oklahoma Speaker Association friends, Dr. Jeff Magee and John Irvin—thanks for your many encouraging words. Thanks, too, to Dr. Nanette Lane, Jean Kelley, and Charles DuBois. Your comments and feedback were so valuable.

I am so appreciative to my good friends, Brenda Richards, Veronica Hurdelbrink, and "Armadillo Jim" and Sheila Schmidt for your editorial comments, but most of all your continual friendship, and incredible support.

Special thanks to one of my nutritional mentors, Dr. Michael Dobbins for your input in the nutrition chapter and for your commitment to whole foods and nutrition.

Many thanks to my talented graphic designer, Brandon Sensintaffar and friend and encourager, Lisa Simpson for the outstanding typesetting job.

I am most grateful to Lindsay Roberts—I thank God for you and all you continue to do to get the word out about health and nutrition.

Many thanks to my Pastors Eastman and Angel Curtis. You are such living examples of motivation and encouragement! Thank you for believing in the gift in me.

Most of all, I thank God, without Whom I am nothing, and can do nothing.

About the Author

Author and motivational speaker, Lorrie Medford has a BA in Communications and is a licensed Certified Nutritionist from The American Health Science University. She also holds certification as a personal trainer from ISSA (International Sports Science Association). She serves on the Board of Directors for the Society of Certified Nutritionists, and is a member of the Oklahoma Speakers Association.

In addition to writing *Why Can't I Stay Motivated?*, Lorrie has written a weight-loss book called *Why Can't I Lose Weight?* and a cookbook called *Why Can't I Lose Weight Cookbook*. A health researcher and journalist, Lorrie has studied nutrition, whole foods cooking, herbal health, fitness, and motivation for more than 20 years. Lorrie taught her weight-loss class at a local junior college and with her own business for more than 10 years, and has taught natural foods cooking classes in Spokane, Washington and Tulsa, Oklahoma for more than 5 years,

She shares her knowledge not only in this book, but in her seminars, and through her nutritional consultation practice, *Life Design Nutrition* in Tulsa, Oklahoma.

Lorrie is uniquely qualified to write about health and fitness. She knows what it's like to be a *cranky calorie counter* obsessed with foods, dieting, and striving to be thin. After struggling with her weight for many years, Lorrie lost more than 35 pounds and has kept it off for more than sixteen years by following the ideas presented in this book.

Lorrie has a rich history of community involvement teaching nutrition and is a sought-after speaker for civic groups, churches, hospitals, and wellness organizations.

You Can Win the "No-Belly" Prize!

I was browsing through the summer issue of a women's magazine which was flooded with advertisements of pretty girls in skimpy swim wear. It was the summer of 1978, and I felt like a fat blob. I found myself wishing I had lived at the turn of the century when even at the beach the ladies were fully clothed! Those long-legged, wool bathing suits hid everything—cellulite, saddle bags and love handles. Today, swim suits are so small they can make even the skinniest girls look fat.

As I looked at those advertisements, the discouraging thought came to me, "I'll *never* look like that. I'll *always* be fat."

When I was about 35-40 pounds overweight, I felt doomed to live with flabby arms and fat thighs. I often gave up hope. I couldn't see myself thin. I remember looking at my thighs and thinking that they would always be fat. I would diet and pounds would come off, but in a matter of months I'd regain everything I'd lost. Change seemed so difficult. Almost impossible. But I later learned that it's *never* over—there's always a way!

I did not stay fat! I lost weight and kept it off. Today I think differently; I see myself differently. I *did* change and you can too.

I meet with thousands of clients every year. And many people lose weight easily from the first appointment. But not every client I've seen loses weight easily. Obviously, teaching them about nutrition and exercise isn't enough. Why not? What's holding them back? Why is it that for some people change is easy and for others it's difficult? Why can't they get motivated and achieve their goals?

A Changed Life

Let me tell you about a young woman from Buffalo, New York who was married at 21, but found herself divorced seven years later. She became trapped in a dead-end secretarial job that didn't match her gifts or talents. She was overweight, with no goals, and no formal education. But she wanted desperately to change. She tried to change, but felt out of control. Shy, depressed, and lacking confidence she took classes and seminars about how to change her life. Delivering her first speech in a Toastmaster's meeting, she was so scared that her knees literally knocked! She married a second time, which only lasted 3 years, but that marriage moved her across the country to the Northwest.

She began a search for ways to become motivated to lose weight and her compulsive behaviors, and spent her time and money over a ten-year period studying nutrition, how to change, and motivation. Finally, at age 34 she received her college degree. She had a dream of speaking and writing books. By now she had lost her weight, became a Christian and attended a two-year Bible School.

For the next seven years, she taught a class at a local junior college. Following that, she became a Certified Nutritionist, and several months later, a Certified Fitness Trainer. Fifteen years passed between the day she received her first degree and the opening of her own business. She became an author at age 51. I know this person well because this person is me!

In my first book entitled, *Why Can't I Lose Weight?*, I talk about the physical causes of obesity, which includes poor digestion, cravings, and sluggish metabolism. I know about all of these because I was an unsuccessful, cranky calorie counter. I have lost weight and kept it off for more than 16 years now. I learned how to get a vision, set goals and change myself and my life. But my journey with weight loss coincided with a journey to find my purpose in life and change myself on the inside.

Today, I have a thriving practice, no weight or health problems, and I have won the "no-belly" prize after all. More than that, I am living my dream! I finished writing drafts for four books in that time; I became stronger and healthier, and I designed my life as a nutritionist, writer, and speaker.

You're So Lucky!

People meet me now and think that I am just lucky because I have a job I love, or my weight loss must have been easy, not like theirs. They have more weight to lose—I only had to lose about 40 pounds. Or, they see the cover of my first book, and think, *What does she know about being over-weight?* Well, as a former compulsive overeater who had a bad self- image, I unfortunately know too much about it!

But it never was a matter of luck. I'm just like everyone else. If I kept eating the same way I used to eat, I'd still be overweight. If I kept thinking the way I used to think, I'd still be overweight. If I hadn't found some tools and skills along the way which helped me to get motivated, I'd still be that same unhappy secretary. I learned how to change and how to motivate myself.

So this book is about changing, getting motivated and really doing it this time. This book contains the material that I taught for seven years in a weight-loss motivational class at a local junior college. It has helped many people to change, and it will help you, too. The emphasis is on motivation for weight loss, but these principles will apply to any project. I used the same tools for change in designing several areas of my life.

Make it a Lifestyle

In my first book, I said that to lose weight permanently requires two things:

1. Discover what's been hindering your weight loss.

2. Make it a lifestyle this time. A healthy diet, along with healthy eating patterns, needs to become a lifestyle—a way of life.

Sounds easy, doesn't it? I mean, pick up any magazine and the cover story will promise quick, easy and painless weight loss as you eat the foods you love! Right, and Elvis is still alive, too!

I know how hard it is to change! Not only have I changed myself and my habits and lost the weight, but I help people make changes daily. The reality is there is a lot of work involved between the initial excitement and hope of a good eating/exercise plan and the day-to-day walking it out.

What Are You Going To Do?

What do you do when you get discouraged? bored? tired? What do you do when you don't feel like you want to go one more day? Or when you just want to give up?

Read this book! Get a strong foundation for change. Know what you are changing and why. You won't be one of those 95% of people who after they lose some weight, gain it all back again. Yes, you will still need some self discipline, but you already have that!

This book is about changing yourself on the inside; changing your thoughts and changing lifelong habits. It's about designing your life for change, and changing yourself from the inside out. That's why I call my practice, Life Design Nutrition.

Where Do You Need Help?

Broken into two parts, this book presents eight steps for successful weight loss. It shows you what to do, why to do it, and how to do it.

Part One is about the mental side to change, and developing healthy habits as a lifestyle. I call it the Life Cycle of Fitness. The steps include learning about change, understanding your thoughts and how they affect your mind and body, finding your motivation, and learning how to set goals and manage your time and life.

You will learn:

1. How to form healthy habits
2. How to change your thinking about diet, exercise and your self-image
3. How to get and stay motivated
4. How to set goals and manage your time and life

Part Two is about the physical side giving you action steps which tell you what fat-burning foods to buy, how to start an exercise program, and how to eat the right amount at the right time. It also includes information on keeping a food diary and knowing about food triggers.

You will learn:

5. How to eat healthy, fat-burning foods
6. How to start and stay with an exercise program
7. How to eat at the right time
8. How to eat the right amounts for you

You Are Already Motivated!

A vital aspect of weight loss is motivation. I didn't always feel motivated, and I used to look for ways to motivate myself. So I would write motivational statements and keep them in front of me.

Throughout this book, you will read dozens and dozens of motivational statements, especially in Chapters 7 and 8. In every chapter you will get additional reminders that you can make it this time, that you have what it takes, that it is possible to change, and that you are going to make it!

As in my other book, I have also written motivational statements at the end of each chapter to encourage you along the way. A summary of these motivational statements is in the Appendix.

You Can Lose Weight!

Perhaps you can identify with the struggles I went through. I loved God. I prayed. I was faithful to live right, but I was still trapped in bad habits I really didn't want to do—such as overeating. But I learned that we may love God and pray daily, but still be missing the practical steps of exactly how we can change. That's why I wrote this book. It's really the book I always wanted and needed. It's about designing your life so that you can change yourself from the inside out.

You can change your habits! You can change your body, your thoughts and your life. Circumstances can change. Things don't have to stay the way they are. You can get so much more out of your life. Life can be exciting and so can change. You are designing your own life every day. Why not design it the way you *really* want it?

I refer to myself as a MN, or motivational nutritionist, because motivation is just as important as nutrition and exercise when it comes to change. I want to inspire, encourage and remind you that you can change your life.

It doesn't matter what has happened in the past, and it's never too late! You can create an exciting future. My greatest desire is that this book will really help you change your life, from the inside out!

PART ONE

The Mental Side of Change

STEP ONE

Get a Foundation for Change

Chapter One

Get in the Life Cycle of Fitness

Some time in 1977, I was leafing through my most recent issue of a fitness magazine, when an article grabbed my attention. A woman who once weighed 250 pounds, was now down to 118! The before and after photos were incredible. I might have been overweight, but I certainly didn't weigh 250 pounds. "If she can do it," I said to myself, "then so can I!"

I hurried to the phone and called the local the health club. On the spot, I signed up for their advertised special. My plans for a new car would have to wait.

The next morning, I woke up before my alarm went off at 5:45 a.m. I couldn't be late for my first aerobics class! It was great! I was there with all the rest of the fitness fanatics jumping, pumping and sweating.

Within a week or so, however, I began to slack off. I threw the alarm clock across the room so many times, it qualified for the frequent-flyer program. I went to the health club less and less until eventually I stopped going altogether.

But after a few months of laying off, I started again. And again. I've heard that when you stop exercising and then take it up again, your muscles have to re-learn all the moves. It's true. And my muscles are definitely slow learners!

On and Off, On and Off

I could exercise sometimes or once in awhile. On and off, on and off. I would start an exercise program and then stop. I would start diets and then stop. I bounced back and forth from good habits to bad habits. You'd think that all that bouncing would have burned some fat! We can all dream about losing weight. That's easy. But if you want to change your size, you have to change yourself inside. And that requires action—consistent, regular action, of eating the right foods and exercise, not just sometimes, or once in awhile. I used to eat too much every day for years. So it took longer than a week or even a month to change permanently. To get and stay active, it helps to understand some basics about change. This is the first part of your foundation for change.

My Mom, the Bowling Coach

When I was a little girl, my mother was a bowling instructor. She was a great bowler and carried a high average. I'll never forget how she taught people how to bowl. Sometimes her students would try fancy methods to send that bowling ball down the lane. But Mom would always take them back to their first step. From that first step, she could see where their timing was off, or what other problems hindered their follow-through.

Like Mom was with her bowling students, I'd like to become your "coach" in the game of weight loss. We'll go back to your first steps, get your basics right, and then build each step from there.

Why Can't We "Just Do It?"

There are two cycles in life—a positive cycle and a negative cycle. Everyone has experienced this. You may make a "New Year's resolution" to eat well and exercise in an attempt to lose weight, and it goes well. You're seeing results. But then, around mid-March for some unknown reason, you fall back into a cycle of bingeing and lethargy. Why does this happen? Why can't we move into the positive cycles and stay there? Why do we bounce back and forth?

The reason can be found in the basis of all behavior—that is the God-given ability to form habits. Often we associate the word "habit" with bad things. We speak of "bad habits," but habits can be good! We all have many good habits like brushing our teeth, taking a shower, or always putting the car keys where they can be found. Once a habit is formed, it's hard to break. That's good except for habits like overeating, or eating large meals too late at night. If we do these over and over, we can gain weight. We just need to keep our good habits and change the ones that aren't helping us to lose weight.

I know this cycle of bad habits firsthand. I used to be a compulsive overeater. There was a time when I could eat two or three bowls of cereal for breakfast and look for a snack an hour later! I was addicted to food. For all I knew, my addiction was permanent, or I might have to go through years of expensive therapy in order to change. It wasn't permanent and I didn't have to do therapy. I used the tools in this book to help me change. They'll help you, too.

Habits Have a Purpose

The habit-forming abilities in our lives are there for a purpose. We did them for a reason.

You know how this works. Haven't you ever had a stressful situation, like your car breaks down when you don't have a lot of extra money? So in your stress, you reach for something comforting—like a candy bar. The good taste and possible emotional connection from being soothed with a candy bar when you were a child, help distract you from the stress and even relaxes you. At first, in your mind, chocolate makes things better. For a few minutes, anyway. Instead of making things better, though, it usually makes things worse!

After the temporary high wears off, we now feel worse, and the original problem is still there.

If candy bars meet a need, we repeat the action. When repeated often enough, it becomes a habit. Therefore, the way to stop any *bad* habit is to identify it, break the pattern, and replace it with something else. This method is one of the tools that I'll describe later.

In a similar matter, overeating becomes automatic. An overeater sets a pattern—a pattern of eating too much. But that pattern of behavior began with a simple thought. That thought may have been: *Eating this food will make me feel better.*

And we usually feel better. Again, it's a temporary pleasure. After the good feeling goes, along comes extra pounds, which bring no pleasure at all! But by now the pattern has been repeated and repeated until it has become automatic in our nervous system. We have lost control. Fortunately, we can break bad habits and our emotional connections to them. I did and you can, too.

Help Me Brush My Teeth

And before you get too upset with yourself and the process of forming habits, think for a moment how crazy life would be if we didn't have the ability to form habits. What if every time you had to brush your teeth, tie your shoes, or drive your car, you had to rethink every movement? I mean, we think it's hard to get to work on time now; imagine how much more time it would take us to just get up and get dressed to go to work every day! Thank God that we have this incredible ability to make a brain-body connection with things we do, so we can do them quicker, without even thinking about them.

We Can Change!

Some of the greatest lies are that we don't have a choice, that we are victims of circumstances, and that we are stuck in a permanent rut and that we must stay there. No!

We have the ability to choose a new way. We can choose to eat new foods, think new thoughts, and make new habits. We can change! We can make new brain-body connections. Within each one of us is a God-given ability to change.

You can choose life and the positive cycle. That's exactly what I did—and I lost the excess weight permanently. The key was to do the right things more often than I did wrong things. You'll discover in the next chapter and ones that follow, that you don't have to do it all in a day. But you keep moving forward progressively with small steps. That's what designing your life is all about!

The Diet Cycle

One of the most frustrating types of a negative cycle is the cycle of fad diets. We overeat to handle stress, and then we feel guilty. We decide to go on a diet, and then we feel deprived. After feeling deprived for a while, we cheat on the diet and eat more. Eating more makes us feel worse, so we go on another diet.

The Diet Cycle

Diet

Guilt   **Depression**

Binge

Food makes us feel good—temporarily. The result is temporary weight loss. We always regain what we lost because we haven't changed our thoughts or what we eat.

Two Reasons Why

Why did we even get in the Diet Cycle to begin with?

Personally, I found two reasons: 1) I wasn't taught how to eat foods that work with, not against how my body burns fat, or that helped me eliminate sugar, chocolate or carbohydrate cravings. 2) I wasn't taught how to take advantage of how our brains form habits to form new healthy habits.

The Life Cycle of Fitness

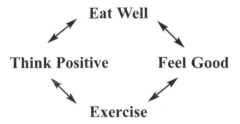

The Life Cycle of Fitness

In the Life Cycle of Fitness, we feel good about ourselves. Health and fitness are a way of life. We don't need food to feel good. We feel good about ourselves and that helps us to form good habits, like eating healthy food and exercising.

I used to let sugar make me feel good, but it ended with the sugar blues, and slow weight loss. I learned to eat foods that made me feel great and helped me lose weight. After awhile, sugar was no longer an issue. It still seems amazing to me that I can walk by pastries and rarely ever want them. On my 50th birthday, my friends had to motivate me to try to eat a piece of my birthday cake! Throughout this book, I share everything I've learned about breaking into the Life Cycle of Fitness.

Once you break free from the Diet Cycle over into the Life Cycle of Fitness you'll eat better, which results in higher energy levels. When the energy levels increase, you'll feel more like exercising. Once you begin exercising, you feel so well physically you'll then feel well emotionally as well. When you feel well emotionally, you'll think positively. Thinking positively enhances your desires and abilities to continue to exercise and eat healthy foods. Hey, this sounds like a good thing!

The goal of this book is to guide you to live in the Life Cycle of Fitness all the time. Of course, everyone may occasionally fall away from their healthy eating plan. (No kidding!) The trick is to get back in the Life Cycle of Fitness quicker, or as quickly as possible. It gets easier every time.

Let's move to chapter 2, and see how we can make changes easier.

Chapter Summary

- There are two cycles in life—the Diet Cycle and the Life Cycle of Fitness. You can choose new thoughts and create new habits.
- Habits are not all bad. Each of us can break bad habits by identifying them, confronting them, and replacing them with good habits.

Motivational Statements:

I can change my thoughts, my habits and my life. I can get and stay in the Life Cycle of Fitness and make health and fitness a way of life.

Chapter Two

Change Is Easy

The first time I ever tried to lift weights, it was fun and easy. For about a minute. Then reality kicked in. My trainer was encouraging me to give him just a few more repetitions. I did, lifting as much as I could. Then, he said, "One more." I thought, *One more? Are you crazy? I barely got up this morning, and I've already been on the treadmill for 20 minutes. I've already expended my muscle strength with just this one exercise, and you want more! This "getting in shape stuff" is hard work!* No one ever told me this. In the magazines, all of the beautiful, long-haired, tanned women are smiling as they lift weights. I remember thinking, *This is hard. It's too much work. I don't know if I can do this.*

How About You?

Have you ever said or thought anything like this:

"I'll always be like this..."

"I'm too old to change..."

"I can't exercise..."

"I can't imagine myself looking any different than I do at this moment."

These are comments taken right out of my journal! I wrote these comments before I understood the process that leads to change. It's not that I didn't try hard enough. It's not that I didn't try good things. Like many other people, I tried dozen of diets and ordered subscriptions to the latest health and fitness magazines. I even bought new sportswear. I traded my gray sweatsuit for a hot pink one. I wanted to sweat in style!

But until I understood more about the reality of change, I was stuck in the Diet Cycle.

I'm Really Stuck!

Last winter, we had a terrific snow storm. Everything was closed. We were all stuck at home. After a few days, the snow started to melt. Looking outside I thought, *I'm from Buffalo. I grew up driving in snow, and I have front-wheel drive. I can get around.* So I decided to try to go to the store. I drove my car out of the garage, but I got stuck in the snow. I sat there, spinning my wheels, and my car wouldn't move. I guess the front-wheel drive couldn't get me out of this one! The more I accelerated, the worse the situation became. I realized that my car would stay right there on the snow until two things happened.

I had to understand what's going on. (As if a woman can ever understand anything that's going on with her car!) I needed to get out of the car and assess the situation. How deep were the ruts? What would it take to get the car moving?

Second, I had to take action or the car would never move. (Unless I wanted to wait for the spring thaw.) Did I need to call Triple AAA? Should I phone a friend? I needed someone to help me get out of the ruts. I knew if I could just get out of my driveway, I could get onto the highway where the streets were plowed.

A few moments later, my neighbor came by and pushed my car right out of the ruts. I was grateful to my neighbor who helped me get on the highway. I thought, *That was all I needed—just a good push.*

Where Are You Stuck?

In this same way, we get bogged down in our bad habits of overeating and making bad food choices. You may have been spinning your wheels thinking you were doing the right things, buying the right clothes and sports equipment. Yet you're still stuck in the Diet Cycle. Americans spend billions of dollars a year on diet drinks, athletic clothes and foot wear. And these things can be steps in the right direction, but sometimes we need more information that will push us back on the highway or in the Life Cycle.

Are you continually losing and gaining the same 10, 20 or 50 pounds? Isn't this discouraging—especially when all that we've really lost are patience, time and money?

Everyone can change. So why is change so difficult? Why do we spend years spinning our wheels, seemingly going nowhere? After working with thousands of people, I've found four main reasons.

Why Does Change Seem Hard?

1. We Don't Know *How* to Change.

What happens when you try to do something that you don't know how to do? You feel frustrated, angry, and may even give up. Many of us have attempted things that we thought were right, but we didn't get the results we wanted.

For example, most overweight women try quick weight-loss diets that will never work. When people follow a low-calorie diet, their body gets efficient at storing fat. After they stop dieting, they get fatter, quicker. Change was temporary, because they didn't know how to eat.

What We Didn't Learn in Kindergarten

We are rarely taught how to eat properly. So most of us are still unknowingly eating foods that make us hungry and store fat. We work against our body's natural responses to foods. Chapters 12-17 will show you what and how to eat.

We are rarely taught about how our brains work to create habits. We often work against this incredible brain-body connection by thinking wrong things about our body and weight while we try to diet and exercise. Eventually the bad habits take over unless we change the thoughts, too.

Be encouraged that the ideas presented in this book will show you exactly *how* to change. For most of us, we need to put action to our faith; that's our foundation for change. In chapters 4-6, you will learn *how* to change the limiting thoughts and habits that hold you back. In chapters 7 and 8, you'll learn *how* to get a vision for change, which is vital. In chapters 9-10, you will learn *how* to use goal setting and time management tools, and finally in chapter 11, you'll use my Life Design Planning Chart to help you make a habit stick. Chapters 12-17 will show you what to eat, and how to exercise.

2. Change Can Be Uncomfortable.

Lifting 50-pound weights is difficult, and uncomfortable! So is not eating desserts, and giving up your favorite foods, especially when all of your skinny friends are still eating them.

If you're sitting down, cross your legs together. Notice how it feels. One leg slipped over the other without much thought. Now uncross your legs and cross them again, only this time, put the opposite leg on top. How does this feel? For most people, it feels different or uncomfortable. One way is no different, or no better, than the other.

When we form a habit, we make new brain-body connections. We get used to doing something a certain way, so it feels strange or uncomfortable to change. Avoiding discomfort is a strong motivator. We can deny, suppress, and even ignore things that desperately need changing just so we can stay in our comfort zone. Like watching TV when the garage needs sorting or the oven needs cleaning. We like things the way they are!

At a recent seminar, my friend Billy Robbins was a keynote speaker. Billy's message was about change, and how, even at a young age, we can get comfortable with change. He told us that even a six-month old child knows how to adjust to new things. After Billy and his wife, Harolronda had their second son, Harolronda told Billy, "You are going to have to learn how to change his diapers!" Billy said, "Fine."

You wouldn't think that it would be a problem, but Billy doesn't have hands. Years ago, Billy had his hands amputated following an accident, and now he has two metal hooks in place of his hands. So when his son saw Billy start to change the diaper, he quickly moved far over to one side, and then again, he moved far over to the other side to help daddy change his diaper. He remembered that the last time he saw those hooks, they were cold! After only one change, he learned how to make a quick adjustment. (Billy now is changing lives and changing diapers!)

A Really Bad Hair Day!

Have you ever been devastated by a bad hair cut? Several years ago, I got a haircut that was so bad, I went out and bought a $90 wig that very same day! I needed something to make me feel comfortable while I adjusted to the change.

Even small changes will require a time of adjustment. A simple change like drinking water instead of coffee, was a giant step for me. When I first made the change, it felt strange and very uncomfortable. It seemed like my car drove automatically to the coffee shop!

When we attempt to give up what may well be a *comfort food,* our bodies cry out, "Wait a minute, this wasn't in the plan!" At that moment, we may decide that it's more comfortable to stay where we are. We don't want to have to let go of the comfortable habits like raiding the refrigerator at midnight, or eating everything on the dinner plate even when we're full because we paid for it *all*.

You Can Do What It Takes

In order to get the results we want, we can make new habits. Because we're so motivated to avoid discomfort, I've tried to make change as easy as possible and to supply you with the tools needed for motivation. Let the ideas in this book help you move out of your comfort zone.

You may not like the feeling of sweating during a good workout. You may not want to give up your cup of coffee and sweet roll that you used to eat with your co-workers at morning coffee breaks. This program will show you how to take your eyes off the coffee break and onto the long-range goals for the new design of your life. Soon you will see that the results are worth the sacrifice. Remember, if changing habits didn't require some discomfort, we'd all be gym groupies instead of couch potatoes!

3. Change Isn't Instant

In our society of "instant" everything, we sometimes forget that life is a walk, not a leap. That's why this is a step-by-step, not a leap-by-leap program. You can learn to aim for consistency, not perfection. Sometimes we may not even know that we are making progress because the internal changes are not always visible, so give yourself time for change.

The day I realized that I was actually waiting until I was hungry to eat—as opposed to eating all day, hungry or not—I was amazed! I couldn't tell you the exact moment it happened. But it's through faith and patience that we inherit the promises—slim thighs and trim tummies!

Take it slow and understand that changing thoughts, habits and behavior will occur progressively. It takes at least a month to make a new brain-body connection. For most people, it took awhile to become 50 pounds overweight. It's unrealistic to expect fifty pounds to come off more quickly than it was put on. I've had clients tell me, "It's been a month and I've only lost 6 pounds." Never mind that it took 10, 20 or 30 years to put the weight on!

You're Not a Failure!

They're used to seeing unrealistic ads for quick weight loss that promise you will lose 40 pounds in 2 months, so they feel like a failure if they didn't lose weight that fast. When people lose weight that fast, they are not losing fat! They went on some type of fad diet or thermogenic that temporarily caused them to lose water weight and some fat and muscle. Follow them for a few months. My experience with thousands of clients is that the quicker they lose it, the quicker they gain it back.

There are dozens of quick, instant methods for weight loss out there, but they don't work and many are dangerous. Taking a thermogenic, "metabolic lift" type product will never replace designing your life and creating new habits, eating better and exercising regularly.

After years of failure, I finally realized that quick and instant applied only to coffee, frozen dinners and credit cards!

If I Can Do It, So Can You!

When I was in my twenties I was undisciplined. But by learning to make small changes, such as walking 15-20 minutes a day and sticking with it, I finally grew to where I actually enjoyed daily exercise. I started walking around my neighborhood. Then I went to an aerobics class six months after that. Finally a year later, I mustered up enough courage to join a health club and hire a personal trainer. And later, I became a personal trainer. If you had asked me to consider lifting weights when I could barely walk around the neighborhood, well, forget it! Never regret small beginnings and changes!

4. We're Not Really Ready

You know when you are ready to change. So do my clients. They know their schedules and what they can and can't do. At the end of an appointment, I've had clients say, "I like what you have said, and I want to change my habits. But I have to wait until I get back from... (a vacation, a wedding, a cruise, and so on.)"

This is a good thing to know! We can plan everything else about our lives, but when it comes to weight loss, we just expect ourselves to be ready. No, there is a time for change. Losing weight is like any other project. For example, would you be ready to clean your garage or run a marathon overnight? No, we need to plan. It's no different when it comes to a major lifestyle change like changing your thoughts, diet, and exercise plan.

You wouldn't paint your house without thinking it through. There are many details to consider—like, who will help you? What supplies do you need? What color paint?

So think about permanent weight loss as a project, and plan when you will start. Most people don't want to waste time or money. If you have a house full of food that you want to use up before you go out and get new food, that's normal.

If you have to clean out the back room, or garage before you can get an exercise machine, or treadmill, that's normal too.

Maybe it's a season where the thought of giving up sweets—like at Christmas time, or family celebrations—

seems impossible. Or it's an extremely busy time like income tax season, or exams at school, and we don't want to take the time and effort required to lose weight—and it does take time and effort!

One More Thing

A word of caution about achieving your goals. Certain things might not happen after you lose weight. For instance, you just lost fifty pounds and that nice-looking guy down the street moved away. Or you lost fifty pounds and no one says anything about it! In fact, your mother, your Aunt Thelma, and your best friend, may still insist that you looked fine before you lost the fifty pounds! Keep realistic goals in mind.

Understanding why change seems hard helps to make it easier. Knowing what to change, that it's normal to be somewhat uncomfortable during change, and that it's not instant, helps. Realizing that we can help ourselves get ready for these changes and approaching it like you would a major household project makes it seem more attainable.

Say, "It's Easy!"

What are you saying about how to change? What you are saying is important, because at some level, our words affect our behavior.

My Pastor, Eastman Curtis, has a motivational slant when he preaches. Several years ago, while he and his wife, Angel were beginning to travel around the country, it seemed so hard for Eastman to get bookings. One day he was frustrated, and he was saying, "Oh, it's so hard." Angel, knowing the power of words, said, "I'm in agreement with everything you are saying. It's so hard."

Eastman realized at that moment that he could be holding back bookings by his own words. So he decided to turn what he was saying around to that it was easy, being in ministry was easy, and getting bookings was easy. Guess what happened? He started getting more bookings. Things were easier. His message was, don't make things harder than they are by saying they are hard; say that change is easy!

You can say that things are easy, or that they are hard. It's your choice. So I want to encourage you to begin to say that with the right approach, change can be easy.

Let's move to the next chapter about discovering what exactly needs to change.

Chapter Summary

- Why does change seem so hard?
  1. We don't know how to change.
  2. Change can be uncomfortable.
  3. Change isn't instant.
  4. We're not really ready.
- Change is easy!

Motivational Statements:

I can change my thoughts to change my size, my habits and my lifestyle. Change is easy and I'm ready to change!

Chapter Three

What Are You Going to Change?

There was a time when the only exercise I got was moving back and forth in the bathtub to mix the hot and cold water! I knew I needed to get more exercise than that! But I also knew that I had to change my diet. I must be eating the wrong foods. And I knew that I had to change my thoughts—see myself differently and all that. And my time—I mean, where was my time going? And I probably had to set goals... Soon, I felt overwhelmed! Again, the thought came, *This is hard! What am I really gonna have to change?*

Different people have different struggles with their weight and health. For Susan, she realized that if she would just quit eating late at night, she would lose weight. Another client named Tony said he needed to eat healthier foods. And still others like Deborah, may need to learn how to find the time to plan healthy meals. I needed to learn it all!

What About You?

I'm a great list maker. I love to make "to do" lists and cross the items off after I complete them. These lists help me stay focused. They help me stay healthy, run a business and write books. When I write everything down, and see it all on paper, I'm not so overwhelmed. I've learned to see what's on the list, and choose to do one thing at a time. Somehow, everything usually gets done, especially the really important things, like paying my taxes!

You're the same way. You write lists and check them off. You can use the same idea to find out what you want to change, and to really figure out where you're stuck.

See, we have to know *where we are* in order to know what to change. Sometimes, without realizing it, we exaggerate where we are. For example, I might say, "I have no control," when in fact I did have some control. I was trying to quit eating sweets. I was walking around the neighborhood several days a week. I was using a Food Diary. One of the best tools I found was to see what I needed to do on paper.

Everyone needs a starting point, or a way to take inventory of where you are and what you want to change. That's what this chapter is about. If you don't have a foundation, I'll help you build one. If you don't have a goal, I'll help you set one. And if you don't know what to eat, I'll help you choose healthy foods.

After working with thousands of people, I've discovered that we usually get stuck in one of any of these eight areas:

1. Get a good foundation for change.
2. Think about the right things.
3. Get motivated.
4. Start planning.
5. Eat foods that burn fat.
6. Start exercising.
7. Eat at the right time.
8. Eat the right amount.

Next, I'm going to list several ideas behind each of these areas. Put a check mark beside the sentence that best describes where you are today. Keep in mind, there are no right or wrong answers here. For people who need it, we're just identifying the specific areas where people get stuck. You can use this information later to help you in the goal setting chapter. In the meantime, I've also given the chapter that will help you to make those changes.

Don't Feel Overwhelmed

Often my clients check several boxes in each group. At the end you will total all the boxes, and start with the top two or three. Don't think about how many checks you have made, because everyone checks several boxes. It's just a tool to know where to begin. Once you establish some good habits in one area, then you can build good habits in other areas.

At the end of every list is one sentence that says that you are already doing this. Check those that apply, too. You may be further along than you thought!

1. Get a Foundation For Change

Do you know when you are in the Life Cycle or how you fall out of it? Your foundation is an understanding of habits and how they change your life. Because change involves habits, we need to know about change. What about you? (Re-read chapters 1 and 2.)

_____ I don't know why I can't stay in the Life Cycle

_____ I want instant results in weight loss

_____ I don't know how to stop fad dieting

_____ I don't know how to change

_____ I think change is uncomfortable

_____ I want change to be instant

_____ I try to change before I'm ready

_____ I am ready to change

2. Think About the Right Things

What are you thinking about? Your thoughts can change your life. So what are you thinking? (Read chapters 4-6 to learn how to change your thoughts.)

_____ I can't imagine myself thin

_____ I can't imagine changing my diet

_____ I can't imagine exercising regularly

_____ I don't feel worthy

_____ I'll change later

_____ I've always been this way

_____ It's too hard

_____ God can help me in every other area except my weight loss

_____ I'm basically unhappy with life

_____ I feel unloved

_____ I feel desperate

_____ I'm afraid I may not get to eat again

_____ I eat for pleasure

_____ I eat out of habit

_____ It's hard to skip meals

_____ I don't understand what triggers me to eat

_____ I have to eat three meals even if I'm not hungry

_____ It's hard to deal with not eating

_____ I'll be tired if I don't eat

_____ I can see myself thin and I believe I can change

3. Get Motivated

Most people really are motivated; they just don't realize it. Check the sentences that apply to you. (Read chapters 7 and 8 for information on motivation.)

____ I don't have a vision of my body at a lighter weight

____ I don't have a plan

____ I don't have a strong enough reason to change

____ I'm too tired

____ I don't feel like changing

____ I don't feel like exercising

____ I can't imagine myself changing

____ I'm already motivated

4. Start Planning

People who fail to plan generally can plan on failing because planning is vital for change. Check the sentences that apply to you. (For help with goal setting, time management and a Life Design Planning Chart, see chapters 9-11.)

____ I don't have any goals

____ I am too busy

____ I don't know how to set goals

____ I don't know where my time goes

____ I never plan my meals

____ I live on convenience foods and diet drinks

____ I'm always too hungry for my meals to stop and think about what I am eating

____ I already have goals, manage my time and/or plan my life

5. Eat Foods That Burn Fat

Check the sentences that apply to you. (If you check even three or more in this list, Chapter 12 on nutrition will help, but you also might want to read my book, *Why Can't I Lose Weight?* which gives the many hidden causes of overweight.)

_____ I crave chocolate

_____ I crave sugar

_____ I drink sodas every day

_____ I buy the wrong foods

_____ I eat out frequently

_____ I eat the wrong foods when I eat out

_____ I don't have any energy

_____ I don't plan healthy meals

_____ I am probably nutritionally deficient

_____ I drink coffee regularly

_____ I have low-blood sugar

_____ I love fried foods

_____ I love sweets

_____ I always skip breakfast

_____ I like processed, artificial foods

_____ I like foods high in salt

_____ I prefer canned foods

_____ I already know how to eat right

6. Start Exercising

Check the sentences that apply to you. Most people are not involved in regular exercise. I wasn't. We didn't grow up with the idea of exercise. For many of us, we have to learn to like it. I want to help you design your life so that you find exercise that you enjoy, and will continue doing week in and week out, year in and year out. (Read chapters 5 and 13.)

_____ I don't want to exercise

_____ I don't know what I should do

_____ I have higher priorities

_____ I'm too old

_____ I'm too lazy

_____ I'm too overweight

_____ I don't believe it's important

_____ It's boring

_____ I don't like doing it alone

_____ I need more energy

_____ It's too expensive

_____ It's too hard

_____ I'm not disciplined

_____ I've never really tried

_____ Other people keep me from exercising

_____ I don't want to be uncomfortable

_____ It takes too much time

_____ I'm too stressed out

_____ I don't like the inconvenience

_____ I can't find anything I like to do

_____ It's too boring

_____ It takes too much time from the family

_____ I'd rather watch television

_____ I already exercise regularly

7. Eat at the Right Time

Check the sentences that apply to you. These are real responses from people in my classes. I was so amazed at when people would overeat. We expect that people might eat at unhappy times, but sometimes they eat during happy times. (See chapters 14 and 15.)

I eat when:

____ I'm bored

____ I'm lonely

____ I'm unhappy

____ I'm happy

____ I'm sick

____ I'm anxious

____ I'm tired

____ I'm discouraged

____ I'm depressed

____ I'm rejected

____ I'm trying to feel better

____ I'm trying to relieve boredom

____ I'm rebellious

____ I'm trying to stay awake

____ I want to relax

____ I want to reward myself

____ I want to procrastinate

____ I'm stressed

____ I want to celebrate

____ I'm around lots of food, like at a buffet

____ I'm watching TV

____ I'm reading a book or magazine

_____ I'm in a car

_____ I'm trying to adjust to change

_____ I'm in a food store

_____ I'm at social gatherings such as birthday parties and holidays

_____ I'm watching a movie

_____ I'm with certain friends

_____ I'm stressed

_____ I'm in social situations, but I'm not hungry

_____ I'm avoiding something

_____ I eat when I'm naturally hungry

8. Eat the Right Amount

There is a perfect amount for you that will keep you healthy and at a good weight. Maybe that extra helping every day is the only thing that keeps you overweight! Check the sentences that apply to you. (See chapters 16-17.)

_____ I eat too much

_____ I am obsessed with food

_____ I don't know when I've had too much

_____ I eat too fast

_____ I eat to please others

_____ Food is more pleasurable than people

_____ I can't help myself

_____ I diet/binge

_____ I only occasionally overeat

_____ I overeat regularly

_____ My parents are overweight

_____ I have to finish everything on my plate

_____ I already eat the right amounts for me

Anything Else?

I've tried to be thorough with what I have found are the top reasons why we get stuck, but I might have missed yours. Right now, write down any other reason why you are struggling with your weight. Finish this sentence: The one main reason why I struggle with weight is_____

_____

_____

_____

Sometimes if we ask the question like that, the most important thing to change pops up out of no where. It may not be on any of my lists, but more than likely I'll cover it somewhere in this book.

Okay, now let's go on to the second step that's about changing our thoughts.

Chapter Summary

Taking inventory of your own personal situation will give you a place to start.

- Get a good foundation for change.
- Think about the right things.
- Get motivated.
- Start planning.
- Eat the right food.
- Start exercising.
- Eat at the right time.
- Eat the right amount.

Motivational Statement:

I know exactly what to change and I expect to succeed.

50

STEP TWO

Get Victory Thinking

Chapter Four

Your Thoughts Can Change Your Life

In the early 1970s, I was living in West Germany. It didn't take me long to discover that I loved their sweets. Wherever we went, I saved room for dessert. In my mind, a meal wasn't complete without eating something sweet like German pastries, puddings or Black Forest Cake. I also gained about 30 pounds fairly quickly! A friend named Kathy gave me some books on diet and health. I began to eat better foods and thought I would try not eating desserts. I remember how I struggled. *Wait a minute. I don't want to do this. Give up sweets? While living here? What was I thinking?*

Now, many years later, I rarely ever eat dessert after a meal. People ask me, "Don't you ever want a candy bar, piece of cake or ice cream?" And my answer is, "No." Why? I changed my thoughts about desserts.

You'll learn the nutritional reasons that motivated me in chapter 12, but in these chapters you'll learn how my own thinking motivated me. Understanding your thoughts and their effect on your life is the second part of your foundation for change.

You Can Believe

All things are possible to him that believeth (Mark 9:23). The Greek word most commonly used for *believe* is *Pisteuo*. *Vines Expository Dictionary* defines *Pisteuo*:

...to be persuaded of, and hence, to place confidence in, to trust. [1]

You are created with the ability to change your thinking which can change your life. Believing in something is called faith. If you think you can do something, you will at least try it. If you think you can't, you won't even try. Not trying reinforces that you can't, but thinking you can at least moves you to action. It's the beginning of every good change! How many things would you have never done if you didn't think you could do them?

If Only I Were Someone Else!

Our ability to change our thoughts is one of the greatest God-given tools we have for changing our lives. Have you ever entertained "if only" or "I can't" thoughts? They go like this:

If only I had... (thin thighs, a thin waist, a smaller size—you fill in the blank...)

If only I had a different body...

If only I was... (taller, shorter, bigger, thinner)

If only I was... (smarter, richer, funnier)

If only I had more money or a better job

If only I was... (good enough, smart enough or attractive enough)

I can't lose weight

I can't change

We'll deal just with self-image in chapter 6. But what about you? Do you entertain these thoughts? Talk about entertaining! Some people open the door, greet the thoughts, and prepare a 5-course dinner for them. They just convince themselves that they just aren't okay the way they are. They need to be someone else. That's entertaining with class.

Change Yourself From the Inside Out!

I once taught a class called, "Your Thoughts Can Change Your Life." I loved teaching that class because the material changed my thoughts, my goals and my life.

Years ago I was overweight, lazy, and unmotivated. I had thoughts like those listed above. I learned that I didn't have to stay that way. I challenged myself to change my thoughts and I changed myself from the inside out. And changing your thoughts can change your life! When we take the time to change these "if only's" to "I can" thoughts, that's when we become "positively motivated."

Many people think that they cannot change. If it were true that we cannot change, then no one would change—ever. But that is simply not true. We're all given the ability to change our thoughts.

Some people just predict and expect bad things for their lives. Guess what they get—bad things. Once when I was watching the weather on TV, the Lord gave me an idea that like the weather forecast, we can predict our own attitude forecast. Here's an example.

John is expecting to be moody today and nice tomorrow. Slight chance of promotion this week. He may experience temperaments flaring with a gloomy outlook for the weekend. Scattered moods throughout Saturday. Frustration predicted. Lots of chance of blues, disappointment and slight risk of depression over the weekend. By Monday, just grumpy and moody.

Then he hears some good news.

Things are looking up. It looks like we can expect promotions throughout the area this week, and by Friday, you can be on top of the world!

That promotion was there all along, waiting for him. It's how he was thinking and what he was expecting that determined his attitude.

What are you expecting? Gloomy days, slight chance of increase? That people don't like you? That life is hard? That you'll never be able to change? Or, that life is great and change is easy?

From Welfare to Millionaire

A man named Peter Daniels proved that a person can change tremendously. Peter Daniels is a third-generation welfare recepient from Australia. He came from a broken home, failed in school, in business, and was illiterate. Many people, including his teachers, his friends, and even co-workers spoke negative things to him. Today, he is a millionaire and a highly sought-after public speaker. In one of his seminars that I attended, Peter said that by reading positive thinking books from the United States, he changed his thoughts. Now he's the author of a number of books, and travels throughout the world speaking in churches and teaching people how to change their lives.

Think about all of the strikes he had against him; a broken home, failure everywhere—he couldn't even read! When I read stories like that, I think to myself, *Okay, what's your excuse, Lorrie?*

Was it difficult for Peter Daniels to change his thinking? Of course it was, but he changed, and so can we!

Have you ever felt depressed about something and then received a phone call bringing good news which cheered you up instantly? Why didn't you stay depressed? What happened? You changed your mind, or your thoughts. You changed your thoughts from "I am depressed," to "Now I'm happy."

Want Some Gum?

Children do this all the time. It's easy to cheer up most children. You distract them to change their thoughts. Just give them a new toy or a stick of chewing gum! You have to use a lot more than a stick of gum with adults!

Changing thoughts was not always easy for me, though. At first, it felt as though I were lying to myself. Do you know how hard it is to declare that you are losing weight when you're standing on the scales and your protruding tummy prevents you from reading the numbers on the scale? Changing my thoughts, along with implementing the other tools outlined in this book, helped me to create new habits which resulted in success and weight loss.

I'm No Longer a Fat Head!

How we think is important! You can be slim on the outside and yet feel fat on the inside. Once I dieted until I got down to 100 pounds. My twin sister, Jackie, told me I looked anorexic. My reply to her was, "But I still *feel* fat!" I had a thin body, but in my head I was still fat. Through prayer and awareness, no longer am I a "fat head." Let's look at a great tool for changing your thoughts.

Your Incredible Computer

We were all designed with an incredible programming device similar to a computer. At a young age, it tells us who we are, and how valuable we are. The information, whether negative or positive, comes from ourselves, parents, peers, teachers, and from circumstances. Everything that happens makes a brain-body connection. I've heard that there are actual impressions, like the grooves on a record that make associations, thoughts and habits in our brains. If we change the association, thought or habit, we can create new impressions. If we can create enough new impressions, long enough, we can change them. But it takes longer than a day! Most people just don't make the changes long enough, or often enough to make permanent change. Two ways to make impressions on your brain are to write them down and say them aloud.

Get a Pen

We are creative people. We are creative, even when we don't want to be.

Here's an example. Let's say you're sitting at your desk trying to write out all the bills that need to be paid. Suddenly an unrelated thought pops into your head such as, "Take out the garbage," or "Go defrost the refrigerator," or "Don't forget to buy toilet paper."

Sound familiar? This is the creative process in action. If you stop a minute, take out a sheet of paper and make a "to do" list, then you can go back to your work of bill writing and the distracting thoughts will no longer bother you. What happened? Writing thoughts on paper helps you take control of them and is more effective than just thinking them. You cooperated with your creative process. You released your mind to concentrate once again on the bills. So I'm going to ask you to get involved with these changes as you work through these three chapters on changing your thoughts.

Here's another example: You're expecting out-of-town guests for the weekend, and you have a long list of things to do before they arrive. (Why does company come right at the time when everything—the carpet, the oven and the refrigerator—

need to be cleaned?) You have so much to do, you feel overwhelmed. But you stop and take the time to write out a list of things that must be done. After they are written down, they no longer appear so overwhelming. You can handle the situation because you can see all the parts.

Write It Down

Writing ideas down helps us deal with thoughts we want to change, too. We need structure. Thoughts in your head are usually scattered and exaggerated like, "I'll never be fit," or "I can't exercise." Until you challenge these thoughts, they usually don't change. When you write them down you can see them, put them in perspective, and change them.

You don't have to be a good writer; just put your thoughts on paper. Rules about spelling and grammar are not an issue. And you don't have to spend hours on this—just a few minutes can work fine. All you need is a pen and paper. Some of my clients like to use bound books with the blank pages and cloth covers. Others are happy with spiral notebooks from the drugstore. Still others use the blank envelope from an old phone bill that was lying around!

Let's go back to the example of millionaire, Peter Daniels. It took a long time for him to change what he believed to be real, and that was his belief that he would always be on welfare. He certainly couldn't deny that his parents and grandparents had all been welfare recepients. He imagined that he could read, write and be successful. Once he faced the limiting thoughts, he changed them, and he changed his life.

You Aren't Limited By Your Past

Some of my eating habits which I blamed on my past were really a result of my bad habits. They were habits I had developed—never mind where they came from. Certainly our past influences our lives, but too many people use the past as an excuse not to change. You can change your life because you can change your thoughts. Once I changed my thinking about food, and I changed my eating habits, the past no longer mattered.

Believe You Can Change

I tried many ways to change, and I believe strongly in the power of prayer. But if praying alone were the answer, you would have lost weight by now. I know. I prayed so much I had holes in the knees of my jeans! Many people pray, but there's more to it than that. We have to change our thoughts, but believe that changing our thoughts will change us, too.

So as with the inventory in the last chapter, we have to know what to change and then we can change it. What follows are five steps that have worked for me that I still use to change my thoughts. If you follow these steps long enough, you can change your thoughts and make new impressions in your brain.

How To Change Your Thoughts

1. Identify It

You need to know what to change. Sometimes it's obvious; sometimes it's not. Put it on paper. Let's give a really simple example.

"I can't resist the temptation to overeat."

2. Think About It

Identify the thought and just think about it. Don't just accept it as true. Think about times when you have been able to resist the temptation to overeat. Here's an example.

"Well, I guess I haven't really tried to resist the temptation. I just assumed that I couldn't. Resisting seemed too hard for me. Maybe I'm not that weak. Perhaps I could if I really tried. Just because I was raised to eat every single thing on my plate, doesn't mean I always have to eat that way. I'm not sure I've really tried. I can resist donuts in the break room; I can resist desserts usually. I probably can resist overeating at night if I think about it, decide to and really try."

3. Forgive If Appropriate

We can be hard on ourselves for being overweight. We're human. We learn by trial and error, not trial and perfection.

Check your heart and see if there is any area where you need to forgive yourself or someone else. If there is no name or face that comes readily to mind, you can skip this step. If you can think of someone or even yourself, then allow yourself to forgive and let it go.

4. Change It

In this step, you write down what you need. Here is where you want to convince yourself or sell yourself on the idea that you *do* have self-control, or you *can* resist, or that you *can* change. Here's an example.

"Wait a minute. I am disciplined. I have God-given self-control. No one is forcing me to overeat. I can take control of my body and what I put in it. I can change the thought that I can't resist to I can resist temptation to overeat. I can find something else to do. I can turn off the TV. I can take a walk, join the YMCA, take my dog for a walk, take a bike ride, and so on. I can change my diet so I'm not as likely to overeat. I can plan my meals. Hey, I can do this!"

5. Write It and Say It

Next, write the new thought that you want, and say it—hear yourself saying it. I've found that if you use both writing and saying together, it works quicker. Here's an example.

"I am disciplined. I do have self-control. I can change. It's all a matter of focus. If I keep thinking I can, then I will begin to believe it. I can change how I eat. I can resist the temptation to overeat."

How To Really Encourage Yourself

If you've been telling yourself limiting ideas for a long time, it will take lots of telling yourself good ideas over and over for at least 30 days to change those thoughts. That's what I did. I had to start by saying and thinking new thoughts, like, *I can lose weight. I can eat right and exercise. Food doesn't have any power over me.*

I'd make a list of the ideas I wanted to work on and think about them and say them over and over. That's how I changed my diet, lost weight and became an exerciser. I convinced myself over and over that I could change. Then I moved to action and making new habits.

I found something that really helped me change quicker. When I was excited and in an "up" time, I made a cassette recording and said things to myself about my life, and my ability to change. Then, later on, when I was depressed and couldn't get a hold of someone to encourage me or talk to, I played my encouraging tape and listened to myself. Within a few minutes, I was encouraged!

Following are a few examples of encouraging statements taken from my own journal. Mark the ones that are meaningful to you. Perhaps you'll want to use them when you make your own *encouraging* tape.

I can change my thoughts and change my life.

I have self control.

I can resist junk foods; in fact, it's easy to resist them.

I can change how I see myself.

Sugar doesn't have any power over me. I don't need candy bars or junk food.

I love fruits and vegetables. I feel great when I eat them.

I love exercise! Exercise is fun.

I can do anything that I want to, if I believe I can do it.

I can exercise regularly and I choose to.

I can resist temptation to overeat.

[1] W. E. Vine, *Vines Expository Dictionary of New Testament Words*, (MacDonald Publishing Company, McLean, Virginia) p. 118.

Chapter Summary

- How To Change Your Thoughts:
    1. Identify it.
    2. Think about it.
    3. Forgive yourself and others.
    4. Change it.
    5. Write it and say it.

Motivational Statements:

I can change my thoughts. I can change my life. I can lose weight. I can be successful.

Chapter Five

Get Off Your "I Can't!"

There's always a good reason not to change your diet, change your thoughts, or exercise! I've heard some great excuses for not exercising over the years, from the weather (too hot, too cold, too wet, etc.) wild dogs in the neighborhood or tornadoes (after all, we live in tornado alley in Tulsa, Oklahoma).

Most of these are ideas that can be challenged or changed. I mean, if it's raining, then why not walk indoors somewhere? We limit ourselves too much.

In the last chapter, we've talked about how to change your thoughts. Now we'll help change them using some examples from some of my clients about changing themselves, their exercise or the food they eat.

There's Always a Way!

Let me tell you about my friend, Jim Stovall. While taking two courses at ORU, he volunteered a couple of hours a day at a school for blind children. They assigned him to a four-year old child named Christopher. They told Jim that Christopher had a cerebral hemorrhage and wasn't able to learn much, but they wanted him to do two things: Keep his shoes tied so he won't trip, and keep him away from the stairs so he won't fall down.

Jim told Christopher, "Before I leave, you'll be able to tie both of your shoelaces, and you'll be able to climb the stairs without falling." Christopher said, "No, I won't." A typical four-year old, Christopher argued like that all day. Jim worked with Christopher. He walked with him. He tied shoes with him. He climbed stairs with him.

Meanwhile, Jim was having his own difficulties. You see, Jim was slowly going blind. He started to think, *I can't do this. I'm not getting any help. I can't cut it.* So he went to talk to the principal of the school for blind children and told her it was his last day, that he couldn't make it in college, and that he was dropping out. So he wouldn't be able to volunteer anymore. Outside the door of the principal's office, Christopher heard every word.

Jim turned away from the principal and saw Christopher who said firmly, "Yes, you can." Jim said, "No, I can't." Again, Christopher said, "Yes, you can."

A Major Turning Point

Christopher challenged Jim to change his thoughts. In his book, *You Don't Have to Be Blind To See,* Jim wrote, "And it hit me just as hard as if I'd run into a wall at full steam: Stovall, quit lying to this kid, and tell him the truth that he can't tie his shoes or climb those stairs. Or prove to this kid with your own life that a person can overcome obstacles and make it through tough times."

Christopher was seven years old when Jim graduated from ORU with an A average. Jim could only see well enough to see Christopher tie both shoes and climb three flights of stairs. Christopher died later that summer. To date, Jim has shared that story with more than a quarter of a million people. Christopher changed his life; and indirectly changed the lives of thousands of people.

I cry every time I hear that story, and I'm so grateful for little Christopher who encouraged Jim to try. To not give up. To believe that he can change. Jim is an Emmy Award winner, a Gold Medalist Olympian, President of Narrative Television

Network, and author of several books. He's now fully blind, but he still speaks to hundreds of thousands of people every year telling the story about Christopher.

You Can Overcome

I have another friend named Billy Robbins whom I mentioned in chapter 2. Billy is president of Jubilee Enterprises in Broken Arrow. An incredibly popular and successful motivational speaker, Billy travels all over the country speaking to organizations about safety. An accident in 1980 left Billy with a double amputation of both hands, and he now has two metal hooks. Can you imagine living life without your hands? An accident like that could have sent Billy into deep depression or even suicide. Billy could have given up, but when he was in the hospital room, he made a choice. He decided not to give up. He decided to make the most of his life. The theme for his speaking business is "Hooked on Life!" He has impacted hundreds of thousands of people with his positive attitude and testimony. His inspirational message is that no matter what your situation, you can still win.

What's Your Excuse?

What about you? You probably don't have to overcome anything like my friends Jim or Billy. But yet there are still thoughts that need to be challenged. Everyone has an excuse for not changing. But for every excuse I bet I could find a successful person who has overcome in spite of that excuse! We can't let excuses hold us back.

I've had lots of excuses about why I couldn't lose weight, or be successful. My first excuse was that I didn't have a computer. I decided to save the money and get a good computer. Then I didn't have the time. I decided later to make time to write. Then I didn't know if I could write well enough.

I decided to just try to write. Then I wasn't sure if I knew enough to write about! That's really silly because I had been studying nutrition for more than 15 years by then. And after I started my nutritional practice, I found even more things to write about.

Face Your Fears

I wrote manuscripts for four books. But deep inside me, there was one more excuse—fear. I was afraid to be published. I loved writing and felt that I had something in my heart to say. But I was afraid of the future—how will my life change? What if I had to be on TV? What if I made a fool of myself on TV? Well, I've been on TV a dozen times now, and it was really fun! Sure, I was a little nervous, but not nearly as nervous as I imagined.

I had to face every aspect of my fears. Through identifying, and then confronting my excuses and fears, I learned to ask, "So what if I make a mistake?" And I've learned to change my focus from myself to others. What great things might happen if this book is published? What kind of impact will it make on someone's life?

A short time ago, a woman named Janice came to my office because she had seen me on "Make Your Day Count" with Lindsay Roberts and Cheryl Salem. Janice cried during her entire first visit. I kept assuring her that I could help her, and at the end of the appointment she told me that she was planning to kill herself if I didn't have any answers for her. I was so happy that I had many answers for her chemically-unbalanced body! Two days later, she sent us flowers, and two weeks later, she was back to work. Her husband came in for an appointment following that and thanked us saying that he had his wife back again. One woman's life was changed because I faced my fear of being on television! Don't let fear be an excuse for not losing weight, or not changing your life.

Top Three Excuses

Here are some of the top three excuses I've heard from clients why they can't change themselves, their diet or exercise. Perhaps you'll identify an excuse you've used in the past and this chapter will help you to get off your "I can't." But don't stop there. What else have you been putting off because you haven't changed your thinking about it yet? Let these examples help to move you in a positive direction no matter what it is you want to change.

Three Excuses For Not Changing

1. I Can't Do It

Convince yourself that you can.

Who says you can't change? You? Your spouse? Your parents? Past failures? Have you even tried?

The first time I tried weight-lifting exercises, I was overwhelmed. The only remote thing I had done was lift a pound cake! I remember thinking, "How did Adam and Eve stay in shape before weights were around?" It took me a whole year before I would even try an aerobics class. I started walking around my neighborhood. Slowly, at first. If I did fifteen minutes, it was a major victory for me. Then I worked up to the aerobics class. My first aerobics class was a laugh—I was so uncoordinated, it was embarassing! When I finally could keep up, I'd trip over myself. Later, I had the nerve to join a health club. I noticed that everyone at the club was in shape already! (I used to wonder where all the people were who really needed to be at the health club.)

You already know that I moved on and became a personal trainer. But where would I be now if I had given up, or if I had said, "I just can't do it?" Probably still overweight and depressed!

Say to yourself:

I can change! I can change myself. I can change
my diet. I can exercise. It's not too hard to change. In
fact, change is fun! I welcome change in my life. I love
the feeling that exercise and good nutrition brings.

2. I'm Too Overweight to Exercise or Eat Better

Convince yourself that you are not too overweight to
change. Being overweight is not a barrier, it only means you
have to choose an exercise you can do comfortably. And your
weight has nothing to do with your ability to eat better.

Start with the easiest, most natural exercise: walking. (See
chapter 13 on exercise for more help.) Choose clothes that
you are comfortable wearing. Who says you have to wear
skin-tight workout clothes when you exercise? When I first
mustered up the courage to begin walking in my own neighborhood, I wore an old blue nylon, loose-fitting, sweat suit. I
was too embarrassed to even wear a pair of shorts. Find good
shoes that fit, too, and make small changes. For example, start
walking for 10-15 minutes, 5 days a week and do it for a
month.

Say to yourself:

I can find an easy exercise that is perfect for my
weight. I don't have to beat myself up to get in shape.
I can start where I am and move forward. I can make
small changes in my diet today. I can enjoy exercise
and I can eat properly.

3. I'm Too Old to Change

Convince yourself that you're never too old to change.

If you think that being older means you can't exercise or
even try new things, tell that to the 80 year-olds at the gym.
Or the group who get up at 6 a.m. and walk in the shopping
mall. Better yet, tell this to the 120-year old men who live in

Pakistan who still farm and live a vigorous, physical life with great health! Who ever said we were too old anyway?

No one is too old to begin an exercise program or to make healthy changes in diet. Whatever age you start exercising, there are positive benefits. If you can walk easily, it's not too late. If you have problems such as aching joints, see a nutritional counselor or doctor who can help you to where you feel like exercising.

Say to yourself:

> *I'm not too old to change. Old is a relative term. The better I eat and the more I exercise, the younger I feel. In fact, I love walking.*

Three Excuses for Not Exercising

1. **I Hate Exercise**

Convince yourself that you love, well, at least like exercise.

I know the feeling—you just don't want to. You feel so lazy that you turn on the television and watch *It's a Wonderful Life* for the twentieth time because you're too tired to hunt for the remote.

Thank God, we don't have to live by our feelings. I've learned that I can change my feelings as often and as effectively as I change my clothes.

As I said earlier, there was one time I could never see myself exercising. Exercise wasn't even a part of my thinking, let alone a part of my life. I had programmed myself for failure in this area. But I decided to change my thinking. Now I love exercise. You can teach yourself to love exercise!

In chapter 12, you'll look at possible physical reasons for not wanting to exercise because you may be genuinely fatigued. But for now, I want you to convince yourself that you really want to exercise. Sell yourself on the idea that you want to, that it will be good for you, and that it will be fun. And find something you like! Use all the tools in this book to help you get and stay motivated.

Don't just sit there. Do something! Put on your jogging outfit and take a brisk walk around the block. Break out of the blahs with action.

Say to yourself:

I do feel like exercising. In fact, I love exercise! It's not a hard thing—it's easy! I feel better every day.

2. Exercise Is Boring

Convince yourself that it doesn't have to be boring.

First, get a partner. Exercise is really fun if you do it with someone else. Or enjoy doing it alone. You might consider getting a tape recorder with earphones and listening to music, humor, or a worship tape as you walk. (See chapter 13 on exercise for more tips.)

After I kept my journal for a time, I noticed something about my exercise patterns. I'd do one thing for a few months and then get tired of it. For example, I'd play racquetball daily for about six months, and get tired of that. Then I'd spend a few months jogging at a local park. From there, I would switch to aerobics. I never seemed to stay with the same routine. Finally, I realized that variety is good for me, so now I plan my schedule for variety.

What about you? Everyone is different. Having seen thousands of clients, I've observed that no two people enjoy the same foods. It's the same for exercise. Find something that you really like and make it fun.

Say to yourself:

Exercise doesn't have to be boring. Exercise is fun! I love the variety and I believe I'm doing the perfect exercise for me. I don't mind exercising alone. Exercise is fun with or without friends.

3. It Takes Too Much Time to Exercise

Convince yourself that you have the time, and it's worth the time.

I used this excuse for awhile. But when I took the time to work out and eat right, it actually saved time. I no longer needed naps. I spent less time being sick. And, best of all, I was no longer depressed due to being overweight and out of shape. My high-energy levels allowed me to accomplish more in a day than I ever had before I started exercising.

Read the time-management principles and life planning chart presented in chapters 10 and 11 so you can figure out what needs to happen for you to have regular exercise. Even if you exercise 90 minutes a week (three 30-minute workouts), you will be making a difference in your body and health.

Find an activity that is close to home that you could walk to or drive to. Or do something easy in your home (workout videos, mini trampoline, jump rope). The best time might be in the morning; then it's out of the way and your evenings are free.

If you regularly schedule one-half hour for exercise for yourself daily, soon you will consider exercise as important as brushing your teeth!

Say to yourself:

I have time to exercise. It's important to me. In fact, I make time. It's worth the time it takes to exercise.

Three Excuses for Not Eating Better

1. I Can't Give Up .... (Coffee, Sugar, Soda, Etc.)

Convince yourself that you can give it up!

One of my mottos is, "Everyone is working on something!" For example, one client named Mary Ann can't give up sugar; while Karen says she can't give up soda. And Frank needs his coffee. First, I have to sell them on the idea of giving it up by explaining that all of these—sugar, coffee and soda work against weight loss. The advantages to any of these stimulants obviously is increased energy, they make us feel good, and they taste good. But there are really more reasons why you should quit than reasons why you shouldn't: they make you gain weight, they mask a real nutritional deficiency, they upset and aggravate digestion, they crowd out nutritional foods, and so on.

Getting off stimulants is hard to do. Why? Most people are so tired that they need something to keep them productive. But one cup of coffee becomes two cups, and so on. The solution is to start weaning and get a healthy alternative for energy, like the B vitamin complex, or bee pollen.

And let's not forget the headaches! Yes, there may be a temporary discomfort. You may feel bad for a couple of days. Convince yourself in the long run, it's worth the pain. That you want to be healthy and fit, more than you want to eat junk food or drink coffee, tea or soda.

But you have to allow yourself to consider the change. Eating candy, cakes and cookies is the American way, but eating too many of these foods is keeping us sick and overweight.

Say to yourself:

I can give up (coffee, tea, soda, sugar). I am willing to at least wean off of these. I have done it

*before and I remember how much better I felt. Weight
loss was easier. Exercise was better. This doesn't have
to be hard. I can do this. I want to be healthier more
than I want to keep eating sugar or drinking coffee,
tea or soda.*

2. I Hate Eating Fruits and Vegetables

Convince yourself that you can enjoy eating good food
like fruits and vegetables. You can't have it both ways. You
can't have junk food and health at the same time. It's one or
the other. What you will find, however, is that the healthier
you eat, the less you will have a desire for junk food! Those
cravings will mysteriously disappear. I have clients tell me
every day that they lost the taste for sugar, coffee, or soda.
Why opt for artery-clogging, diabetes-producing foods when
you can choose energy-giving, health-promoting foods? Why
not begin to change those unhealthy thoughts, too?

Say to yourself:

*I love and enjoy good foods. I love fresh fruits and
vegetables. I love what good foods do for me. I always
feel better when I eat better. Junk food is a thing of the
past. I am no longer willing to sacrifice my health for
the taste of processed foods.*

3. It's Too Expensive to Eat Healthy Foods

Convince yourself that it's not too expensive to eat right.

I know the price people have to sometimes pay to change
since I counsel people all the time. Realize that if you cut out
all of the nutrient-depleted (junk foods), and processed foods,
you will find extra money for more nutritious foods such as
fruits and vegetables! Cutting out coffee, soda, and let's go
even further—alcohol and cigarettes will really loosen up
some change!

Unfortunately, junk food is cheap. It's a shame that real fruits and vegetables, and even frozen foods can cost more. But what is the real price here? The money you spend on good food and whole food nutritional food supplements will some day save you thousands of dollars on heart surgery, or medications for diabetes, or high-blood pressure or cholesterol. I want you to really sell yourself on the idea that you don't need stimulants such as coffee, tea, soda and sugar. Read books like *Sugar Busters* or *Sugar Blues* to help motivate you. Understand what these stimulants are really doing to your body.

Say to yourself:

It's worth the price I need to pay to eat right, plan meals, make better choices when I go out. Even small changes help me get healthier. The better I eat, the better I feel. Eating right can prevent many diseases. I am worth it.

What About You?

Which one of these excuses have you used in the past? What unique excuse do you have that wasn't included here? Get out a pen, write it down, and start to evaluate and challenge it. Then replace it with a better thought

That's all they are—*excuses!* You can change; you're not too over weight, or too old. You *can* exercise! And you can find time to exercise. Find something you like and make it fun! You *can* eat right. You can give up coffee, sugar, soda or tea. You can enjoy eating fruits and vegetables. And you can afford to eat well.

Never Give Up!

Many people quit before they get their victory. They just don't go far enough. When you plant a seed in the ground, it doesn't come up immediately. It takes time for things to grow. Give yourself one, three or even six months to change!

In a similar manner, it takes time for you to change habits, and it takes time for you to change your thinking. Keep on saying what you want, keep on doing what you know is beneficial, and then be patient. Allow for the period of time between planting and harvesting. Never, never give up!

Chapter Summary

- Excuses For Not Changing
  1. I can't do it.
  2. I'm too overweight to exercise or eat better.
  3. I'm too old too change.
- Excuses For Not Exercising
  1. I hate exercise.
  2. Exercise is boring.
  3. It takes too much time to exercise.
- Excuses For Not Eating Better
  1. I can't give up... (coffee, sugar, soda, etc.).
  2. I hate eating fruits and vegetables.
  3. It's too expensive to eat healthy foods.

Motivational Statements:

I can change. I can exercise. I love exercise. I can eat right. It's easy for me to give up foods that hinder my weight loss.

Chapter Six

You Are Good Enough, Smart Enough and Attractive Enough

One morning, while getting ready for work, I put on a brand new dress. It was perfect—the right color, style and fit. When I went out the door to go to work, I felt great. Like I tell my friends, it was a great hair day! Everything went well that morning.

After lunch, I stopped in the ladies' room. It wasn't until I caught a glimpse of myself in the mirror that I saw I had a run in my left stocking, my bangs curled (I hate it when they do that!) and I had some ink on my face! My first thought was, *Now how long has all of this been going on? I look awful!* All of a sudden, I lost my confidence!

I was the same person who left the house full of confidence. Three hours later, I was full of doubts. I had to remind myself that my value was not found in how I looked.

Who Are You?

Let's talk about the most important thoughts you have, and those are the thoughts about your self-image or how you see yourself and your ability to succeed.

Your self-image is often compared to a thermostat that we set. Because we keep that thermostat at a particular level, we continue to perform within a certain range. That means unless we change our thoughts about ourselves, we will stay in our comfort zone. We won't try new things. We won't dare to imagine ourselves slimmer, healthier, or even in a new vocation. We won't try to imagine a better life, or that we can live our dream.

Live To Serve

Why would we work on something like our self-image? I mean, wouldn't it be better if we were spending time helping other people rather than focusing on ourselves? Yes! That's the point. In a perfect world, we would all be so happy with ourselves, our talents, our place of service, our looks and our personality that we no longer need to think about us. We can then live our lives serving others. But so many people can't get to that place because they aren't happy with themselves yet. Rather than help others, they compare themselves to others. So it's worth the time to change yourself inside.

You've no doubt heard the story of how trainers work with elephants. When the elephant is small, a heavy chain is fastened to their leg and then staked in the ground. The elephant learns at a young age that as long as he feels the chain on his leg, he can't go anywhere. Later, a full-grown elephant can be kept in place with a weak piece of rope. A chain is no longer needed. All he knows is that he feels the object around his leg and in his *mind* he can't go anywhere. If that elephant only knew, with one small yank, he could break the rope, he would be free to go anywhere.

We're Smarter than Elephants!

When we are young, we make pictures of ourselves, based on what people say about us. These pictures eventually form our self-image, and unless we change them, we live according to them. If our picture is overweight or unathletic, that's how we'll stay. If our picture is unsuccessful, then we won't try to succeed. The chains of limiting thoughts about ourselves and our ability to change that we experienced in childhood are now just weak pieces of rope. With some effort, we can break loose, change those thoughts and be free.

We all live within the boundaries of our self-image or internal pictures, whether healthy or unhealthy—positive or negative. Our thoughts and even our behaviors come from how we see ourselves. But thank God, we don't have to stay limited by things that people told us as children.

Miss Phillips Was Wrong

Millionaire Peter Daniels wrote a book entitled, *Miss Phillips, You Were Wrong*. What a great title. What a great book. In his book, he took every chapter to explain why Miss Phillips was wrong about him, how she did not have final authority in his life, and how she did not understand him. When Peter was seven years old, Miss Phillips told him, "Peter Daniels, you are a bad, bad boy and you are never going to amount to anything." Peter explained how this event affected his attitude to the point where it became a self-fulfilling prophecy. But he didn't stay that way. He rose above these limitations. He rose above the words of Miss Phillips that he didn't have the ability, or that he would not amount to anything. Why should we let the wrong ideas of other people create our current ideas about ouselves?

You've probably heard examples of how people who were told they would never amount to anything didn't. But you might also have heard inspiring examples of people who were told they wouldn't amount to anything turn that around and become rich and famous, like Peter Daniels did.

What Do You Say About Yourself?

I've had clients who repeatedly said negative things about themselves. However, once I challenged them about it, they were able to stop saying those things, like they couldn't change, or weren't good enough for whatever reason. We often live up to our labels.

Many years ago, I read a book entitled *Psycho-Cybernetics* which was written by a plastic surgeon named Maxwell Maltz Surprisingly, when he removed ugly scars from people's faces, he noticed that it often improved their self-image. But he also discovered that it didn't always improve their self-image! What's up with that? Even though they greatly improved their appearance, they didn't improve their self-image because these people changed on the outside without changing their thoughts, beliefs and attitudes about themselves on the inside.

Many years ago I was invited to speak to a local chapter of an Overeaters Anonymous Group. They invited me to come and share my testimony of how I overcame my habits as a compulsive overeater. I talked about the importance of words, and how we can change ourselves with nutrition and words. (You'll learn more about nutrition and overeating in chapter 12.) I explained that every time I called myself an overeater, I was reinforcing my thoughts, images and beliefs so the actions associated with an overeater would follow.

I told them how I changed my image of myself with words. Instead of calling myself an overeater, I said that I was an overcomer. Instead of labeling myself as a "fat personality," "weak," or "unable to change," I changed my thoughts and words to say: "I am learning how to be free from overeating. I am changing myself and my diet."

I had to see myself differently, and start seeing and saying what I wanted, not that I was an overeater or would be an overeater the rest of my life! I don't believe that calling yourself an overeater is helpful. My message to them was, why keep saying what you don't want to be? Your body responds to your thoughts. You'll get better results if you change it to "I'm an overcomer!"

Your Thoughts Change Your Actions

Here's another example. Toni believes that people don't like her, so she acts on that belief. What does she do? She acts as though people don't like her. Perhaps she's shy or reserved. Because of her beliefs, people don't respond to her well and she perceives that they are acting as though they don't like her. That, in turn, reinforces her original thought that no one likes her. She decides now that people don't like her, and this causes her to act in such a way that people don't like her! Perhaps she's rude or short with people. All this happens because of her original belief.

What would happen if she turned the belief around and just assumed that people liked her? What's the worse that could happen? People would like her, and even if they didn't, at least she's not living a self-fulfilling prophecy that they don't. What are you saying about yourself? What kind of labels do you put on yourself? "Oh, I'm so clumsy!" Or, "I'm a loser," or "I'm a failure."

I believe that self-image can be defined in three important ways; our internal value, our intelligence and our attractiveness. Let's look at three examples.

You Are Good Enough

What makes you feel good enough? I've often asked clients, "What would you have to do to be good enough?" They think about it, and after awhile, they often say things like, "Well, if I lived in a better part of town, or if I made more money, or if I were smart like so and so, I would be good enough."

Think about a little baby. We all come into the world naked. We come with nothing, just this incredible potential that God puts inside all of us. Besides, I believe that God believes we are *all* valuable. He created each one of us special for His design and purpose, and since He gave us what we needed, we have enough. We are good enough. None of those external things really has to influence how you feel about yourself. You know why? We make ourselves good enough by how we *feel* about ourselves. You are good enough when you think that you are! When you believe that God really made someone good when He made you. Having a good self-image is about accepting yourself and enjoying yourself. That's one of the greatest thoughts you can have.

You Are Smart Enough

I was talking to a friend once who said, "I'm not smart enough." I encouraged her to answer some questions. I first asked her, "Who decided how smart you would be? Did you?" She said "No, I'm a Christian and I believe that God made me."

I asked her, "Do you have gifts and talents from God?"

She replied, "Yes, I love people and I have a lot of compassion for them. I enjoy helping people."

So I said, "Do you think that your intelligence is enough for the purpose that God has called you? I mean, God didn't call you to be a bank president or rocket engineer, did He?"

She said, "No. I see where you are going with this. I guess that I don't have the same kind of intelligence as a bank president or rocket engineer. God gave me what I needed."

There will always be people smarter than you. Your intelligence is God given, so in the end accepting yourself and doing the best you can is all that counts.

You Are Attractive Enough

And finally, what makes you attractive enough? I know women who have had all kinds of cosmetic surgery and are still not happy with themselves. Even though they may have made changes on the outside, they still have fears and insecurities inside.

I know other women who don't wear any make up, never had surgery, and are perfectly happy. Who decides if you are attractive enough? You do. You can accept yourself right now, if you want to. It doesn't mean you don't try to be your best; it just means you like who you are. Or as I say, "I clean up real good."

Granted, in America, the land of beauty salons, tanning beds and cosmetic surgery, a person can change almost anything they want. In a day, they can wear different contact lenses, color their hair, and get a tan. Women can change so many things without surgery that it's possible for a husband to come home one day and be greeted by a different woman than the one whom he left that same morning!

I'll never forget that when I was overweight, I had a poor self-image, which was tied to my weight. I decided to dress better. Instead of wearing dumpy clothes, I went to Nordstrom's and bought some new clothes—hot pink tops and stylish suits. I took aerobics classes, even though it was hard for me at times. I ate better. I put these all together and I really began to feel better about myself even though I was overweight. I decided to accept myself as I was instead of waiting until I lost weight. I felt like I was a work in progress and I was valuable.

There will always be someone prettier, skinnier, or smarter than us. Comparison will never end. So in the end, "being the best you can be" is the best advice!

When will you accept yourself? When you lose 40 pounds? When you get married? When you get a promotion, or make more money? When will you be good enough?

Change Your Picture

You have an internal picture of yourself which makes your self-image. You can change it by changing the picture with your own imagination. You do this all the time. When you go to the store to buy a dress, you imagine what it would look like on you. Or you imagine how a new hairstyle might look on you.

So let's consciously create a picture of how you want to be. For example, I *first* had to imagine myself roller blading, or lifting weights. Imagine yourself as a healthy, active person. See yourself doing what you would like to do. Think about how you would look, and how you would act. Think about what your life would be like. What else would you enjoy if you were in that body right now? How would you feel about yourself?

To make it more real, take a pen and make some notes to describe the new you. You will want to use several senses to internalize these words. See them, feel them and say them. I'll give you an example.

1. This Is How I *Look*:

Example: I see myself walking regularly. I enjoy exercise. I see myself slender and attractive. Clothes fit me well. I am attractive enough.

Now you write it: _____   _____

_____

2. This Is How I *Feel*: _____   _____

_____

Example: I feel healthy, attractive and self-confident. I feel great about myself. I am good enough, smart enough and attractive enough.

Now you write it: _____

_____

3. This Is What I *Say* to Myself:

Example: It's easy for me to exercise and eat right. It's okay to look good. I don't have to compare myself with others. I really accept myself. I really enjoy helping and serving others. I am good enough, smart enough and attractive enough.

Now you write it:_____

_____

What you have just created here is your new self-image.

Take whatever you have written and transfer it on three-by-five index cards. Tape them to your mirror, put them on the refrigerator, or carry them in your purse. Carry them with you and repeat them out loud. Especially repeat them just before going to bed at night, and first thing in the morning.

If you do this consistently you will begin to start seeing yourself a new way. You'll catch yourself when you say the old thoughts, like, "I'm too fat," or "I'm too old." You'll say, "No, I'm changing now. I see myself differently. I look and feel great about myself. I'm good enough, smart enough and attractive enough. I enjoy myself and others. I love my life!"

We don't have to stay the same. We can change our self-image. We can program ourselves to always think positively about ourselves. We can consistently visualize ourselves and our lives the way we want them to be.

Chapter Summary

- We make our self-image.
- We can change our self-image and go beyond our comfort zone.
- See it, feel it, and say it.
- Keep the image before you.

Motivational Statement:

I am good enough, smart enough and attractive enough!

STEP THREE

Find Your Motivation

Chapter Seven

Why Aren't You Motivated?

I was thinking about my lack of motivation one day when the thought hit me. *When was I taught to design my life, or how to set major long-term goals for my life? Kindergarten?*

When was I taught how to exercise? I remember trying to get *out* of gym class in school. When was I taught to eat foods that burn fat? I ate what Mom taught me to eat, and she ate what her mom taught her to eat. Well, who taught their moms? And what about our schools? Most schools now have vending machines for soda and junk food. Most TV commercials, magazines and books contradict each other so much that everyone is confused about what to eat!

What About You?

Why aren't you motivated to eat right and exercise? Maybe it's because you grew up in a nation that encourages overeating everywhere you go, like big gulps and all you-can-eat-food bars. Or perhaps it's because you live in a country where we sell soft drinks that things "go better with," but that work *against* how your body burns fat. Or, it might be because we live in a time where real food is harder to find than your friends at the crowded movie theatre.

We grow up with the idea to "live the easy life," and work hard so we can relax, with all the latest modern conveniences. We are encouraged to get a riding lawn mower, so we don't have to exert ourselves so much.

Something To Call Home About

I often wonder what an alien would think about our culture. We eat all day, don't exercise, then read tons of books and spend millions of dollars a year trying to figure out how to lose weight and get fit! Go figure!

We Don't Learn in a Vacuum

We're not motivated because we haven't been taught how to be motivated, or how to design our lives for health and exercise. If you did grow up in a health-minded family that taught you to exercise and eat right, do you think you would have a weight or fitness problem now? Probably not.

Most of us just grow up, eat like our parents, and then at 35 or 40 our lack of knowledge starts to catch up with us. "All of a sudden" we can't eat like we used to. We can't lose weight as easily as we did. Just when we start to get our lives together, our bodies start to fall apart!

Why Else Aren't We Motivated?

Okay, I'm switching back over to my certified nutritionist hat for a moment. For years, I read books, went to seminars and listened to motivational tapes. But sometimes I still didn't get motivated! And I was still depressed! Sometimes everyone around me was excited and I was depressed. Talk about losing motivation!

I've discovered there are several physiological reasons for lack of motivation. In fact, in my office, I deal with these first. My first book covers them in more detail (see *Why Can't I Lose Weight?*) and we'll look at them again in chapter 12, but let's look at them now:

1. Fatigue from nutritional deficiencies. Doesn't it seem logical that if someone is tired, they don't find exercise particularly appealing? Who wants to exercise if they can't get

out of bed? So the first physical reason is fatigue from nutritional deficiencies. These include a B complex, B12, folic acid or iron deficiency. Check with your doctor or a qualified nutritionist.

2. The second goes beyond nutritional deficiencies to hormone imbalance and is fatigue from hypothyroid (low thyroid) or hypoadrenal (low adrenal). Some estrogen hormone products, for example, encourage weight gain, fatigue and depression. Every day I recommend changes in people's diets that can prevent these imbalances so they feel like exercising! You will need to see your doctor or qualified nutritionist for these.

3. Lack of knowledge about how your body works. You may be eating foods that are making you tired, and putting weight on you! (See chapter 12 in this book, and my other book on weight loss for help in this area.)

I Need Motivation!

I've worked with several thousand people in the last 15 years, and in weight-loss classes and counseling, the most common cry for help is motivation. At my last motivation class, when I asked why they were taking the class, one of my clients named Gaye, asked, "Can you give me a pill that will help me get motivated?"

Getting motivated is the third part of your foundation.

I, too, knew all the reasons why I *should* exercise, but that didn't keep me motivated enough to keep on exercising month after month, year after year. I knew why I *should* eat better, but it didn't help me to continue to eat better all the time.

If we could just change without having to deal with our thoughts or habits, it would be easy to lose weight. We wouldn't need more books, teaching tapes, and diet plans! It's easier *not* to do things such as exercising and eating right. It takes energy and motivation to change things. But isn't this true with everything? It takes energy and motivation to attend night school while working full time, or work 10-12 hours a day while you build your business. Changing your life will take some effort, but like the college degree or business success, it's worth it. But we need motivation to keep on going.

So What is Motivation?

The dictionary's definition of the word *motivate* says this: *"To stir you up or rouse you to action."* Motivation then is the drive which moves you. It's energy that keeps you moving. Remember our example of my car stuck in the snow? What I needed was a strong push. That's motivation.

How Do You Get Motivated?

Where do you get motivation? I mean, who really *feels* like exercising the first time when you've gained 40 or 50 pounds? Who *feels* like watching your diet when those old food habits sneak back? Do you ever "just do it?"

Motivation is a process, and it starts in your mind. Remember how you felt when you first started an exercise program? Remember how motivated you were? It's not that you were not motivated; you were. Any time you ever started a diet and exercise program, you were motivated, stirred up, roused to action. You decided to do something, and you set your mind and did it. And you felt even more motivated after you started a good eating plan and exercised. What a wonderful feeling of accomplishment. You got more motivated as you continued.

So remember that motivation and begin again by selling yourself on the idea that changing is more important than staying the same. Set your mind to change. Make a decision to change. Then move into action, and your motivation will get stronger as you go.

People get motivated in different ways. Some people could be motivated by fear of heart or health problems. Some people are motivated by guilt. Some people are motivated by knowledge, such as when you learn what foods actually store fat, you will be more motivated to stop eating them and eat foods that burn fat. Let's keep it simple.

Three Parts To Getting Motivated

1. Get a Picture

Getting a picture of what you want is the beginning of motivation: change, movement, and action. I'm talking about getting an internal picture, (also called imagination), but you may even have a physical picture of yourself at a time when you were slimmer or more active.

What do you want to look like? How fit do you want to get? How many pounds do you want to lose? What shape do you want to be in? What size clothes do you want to wear for the rest of your life? You'll get more help with this step in Chapter 9 on goal setting, but of all the tools I've used, this one is vital because you have to imagine it before it can happen.

Then, when you do something long enough, you develop a habit. And after you develop a habit, you automatically have more self control. But it all starts with that picture. My clients and good friends know that I like Mickey Mouse. I have Mickey Mouse dolls for children to play with in my office, and Mickey office supplies. I have Mickey and Mini dolls over my fireplace at home.

We all enjoyed the Wonderful World of Walt Disney as children. But as an adult, I really admired Walt Disney. He believed in himself, in his mouse character, and in his vision.

Even though people rejected his early mouse cartoon, he kept on. Even though bankrupt several times, he never gave up. He inspires me, and when I look at my Mickey, I am reminded of a man who never gave up! Imagine the number of people he has influenced in the world. He helps children make dreams, and allows people to make their dreams come true.

See It First

I remember getting a picture or image for weight loss. I went out and bought a colorful spandex workout outfit. Yes, I was fat, and no, I didn't go out in public with it on! But wearing it made me feel fit. It helped me. Like putting a picture of my head on a thin model's picture I found in a magazine. I pasted it on the refrigerator door and it worked. It helped me to see myself fitter! Hey, I believe in doing anything you can to move you forward.

Sixteen years ago, I remember getting a picture or image for fitness; I wasn't raised an exerciser. I imagined myself roller blading and lifting weights before I tried them. Later, I learned how to roller blade and lift weights. I remember imagining myself finishing college which I accomplished in my mid-thirties. I remember imagining myself having a book published, and later setting goals to write manuscripts, two of which are published and the other two are ready for publishing. I remember imagining myself teaching classes and later I gave an outline to the director of a junior college for a class that was on my heart. I taught that class nearly seven years!

Sixteen years ago, I imagined myself having a nutritional consulting practice. Being a bookworm, I've read thousands of nutrition books and studied nutrition. After I got my CN, I didn't know how to run a business. So I took classes with the Small Business Association. As far as I know, I was the only full-time practicing CN in the state of Oklahoma. I started in a one-room office, and I did everything from booking appointments to counseling and selling supplements. Today, I'm in a three-room suite, and I have three assistants.

And sixteen years ago, I imagined myself as a motivational speaker. I saw people like Zig Ziglar and Mamie McCullough, and they encouraged me tremendously. The first time I ever spoke in public, my knees knocked! I have been teaching or speaking for more than fifteen years, I speak somewhere every month.

What you picture or imagine, you expect. Things come to people who are using their imagination or expecting things. I don't know how it happens; I just know that it's a God-given tool for change. You get what you are imagining, believing for, hoping for, and expecting to come. So expect good things to happen to you. Expect to change. Expect to be successful!

2. Get a Plan

Having a picture and imagining yourself differently is great. But that's just the first step. Next comes all the work. For example, when I wanted to be a speaker, I found a local Toastmaster's Group and wrote and gave speeches for a total of three years. Attending these meetings gave me knowledge and confidence. Whenever I've had a picture of what I wanted, I researched the best ways to accomplish my goals.

Obviously, I studied nutrition and exercise and used the goal setting and planning tools in this book. What about you? If you are wanting to lose weight, and have a picture or image of where you want to be six or twelve months from now, then what are you going to do? How will you eat? Where and when will you exercise? How will you handle temptation? How will you stay motivated?

This book is packed with tools for keeping you motivated, especially chapter 9 on goal setting, 10 on time mangement and 11 on life design planning. So don't worry too much immediately about your plan, because you will make a plan as you work with this book. This step will keep you in the Life Cycle of Fitness.

3. Get a Strong Enough Reason to Change

Why, why, why should you change? To feel better, look better, get stronger? To reach your fitness goals? Ya gotta wanna! To have to want to lose weight more than you want to stay where you are. That reason, together with knowledge, goals, and belief, stirs you to continued movement and success.

You probably have had strong reasons why you have wanted to lose weight before. I did. Perhaps you wanted to get the attention of someone of the opposite sex. Or, you wanted to lose weight for an upcoming wedding, family reunion, or class reunion. There must have been some strong motivator or reason why you have wanted to lose weight. Whatever it was, you really had to want to enough, or you wouldn't even try. Why spend all of that time and energy otherwise? And it does take some time and energy. So what is your reason?

Why Should I Lose Weight?

If you don't have one, let me help you find one by using an exercise. Below are two lists. One is a list of reasons why you *want* to lose weight. The second is a list of reasons why you don't want to. These lists are made up of responses I've received from students in my weight-loss classes over a ten-year period.

Put a check by the ones that best describe you. (If you have one that's not listed here, add it on the blank lines below.) You may be surprised at the results.

Why Should I Lose Weight?

_____ I'll have more self respect

_____ I'll have more confidence

_____ I'll look and feel better

_____ I'll be healthier

_____ I'll live longer

_____ I'll like my body more

_____ I'll have more energy

_____ I'll be happier

_____ I'll be more attractive

_____ I'll be an example for my children

_____ I'll feel more comfortable in social settings

_____ I'll lower my risk of heart disease

_____ I'll have more fun in life

_____ I'll be able to wear nicer clothes

_____ I'll be more attractive to the opposite sex

_____ I've save money on food

_____ _____

_____ _____

_____ _____

Why Shouldn't I Lose Weight?

_____ I'm tired or depressed

_____ I'm happy with myself right now

_____ I don't think I can do it

_____ I don't know why I should

_____ I don't care

_____ I'm not worthy

_____ I don't want to give up anything

_____ I don't want to be uncomfortable

_____ My life is too stressful

_____ I don't have anywhere to go to work out

_____ _____

_____ _____

_____ _____

Count up your check marks. Which list has more? If you are like most people, you will discover, to your delight, that there are far more reasons why you should lose weight than why you shouldn't!

When I first did this exercise, I had 15 reasons why I should lose weight and only 2 reasons why I shouldn't! What a pleasant surprise to learn that I was more motivated to change than I thought! Let this exercise motivate you!

By the way, if you checked, "tired or depressed," as I said earlier, nutrition will be an issue for you. Don't skip chapter 12! Having more physical energy will enhance your motivation.

Imagine Your Future

Here's another way to get motivated to be healthier by using your imagination. Take a moment and imagine your life if you lose weight and become fit. Imagine the great clothes you will get to wear, the improved quality of your life from getting and staying in the Life Cycle of Fitness. Imagine the friends you will have, and the impact you can have on other people's lives.

Now imagine your life if you don't lose weight, or become fit. Imagine the clothes you will never get to wear, and how life can be if you aren't fit, can't play tennis or roller blade, and don't want to be seen in a swim suit. I remember not being able to play tennis, and not wanting to be seen in a swim suit. This picture never motivated me! I wanted to change, to do what it took to get in the Life Cycle of Fitness. We were designed by God to be active. Doesn't the first picture feel better? Yes, yes, yes!

Let this chapter help you get motivated. Think about the things you might have been putting off that are hindering a higher quality of life. Imagine yourself doing something new, or being active in a way you hadn't imagined before. Imagine yourself in new clothes, and even in a new job, hobby, or new group of people. It's okay to dream, make pictures in your mind, and imagine, because that's the beginning of every significant change.

Now that we know how to get motivated, let's move on to how to stay motivated.

Chapter Summary

- Motivation is an inner drive that stirs us to action.
- Nutritional reasons for fatigue:
  1. Fatigue from nutritional deficiencies.
  2. Hormone imbalance.
  3. Lack of knowledge about how our bodies work.
- Three parts to getting motivated:
  1. Get a picture.
  2. Get a plan.
  3. Get a strong enough reason to change.
- Know why you want to lose weight.

Motivational Statements:

I really want to change. I want to lose weight. I want to look and feel better. I want to eat right and exercise. I want to change more than I want to stay the same.

Chapter Eight

How Can You Stay Motivated?

As a personal trainer, I see athletes every day at the health club. Just looking at them, you would imagine that they love working out. They jump out of bed at 5 a.m. and drive to the gym. They jump on the treadmill for 20 minutes. Then they can't wait to lift weights. Heavy weights. Unlike the rest of the population, they have no problems with motivation. Right?

Wrong. I was surprised, too, that many athletes don't always *feel* like working out. They don't feel like getting up at 5:00 a.m., or driving to the gym. They don't feel like jumping on the treadmill and then lifting weights. Most of them have *learned* to work out. They work out no matter whether they feel like it or not. But they like the way they feel after working out. They have developed a lifestyle around exercise and fitness. They created healthy habits, they got in the Life Cycle of Fitness, and they stay there. If they fall out of the Life Cycle, they get right back in it again.

We've talked about what motivation is, and how it works. You may have even discovered just how motivated you are. You know why you want to lose weight. You know that you have to do the work. You're getting a picture, making a plan, and you know why you want to lose weight. But how long will it last? How can you stay motivated? What are you going to do when you want to give up? How are you going to do it long enough to make it a lifestyle?

Everyone hits a time when they just don't feel like exercising. Or they want to give up altogether. We all experience down times!

But successful people have ways to keep themselves motivated. Here are a few tips that really helped me to press on, stay in the game, keep going on, even when I wanted to quit.

1. Keep Your Picture Before You

Step one for *keeping* motivation is the same as step one for *getting* your motivation. You really need that picture or image before you.

Here's an idea that some of my clients have used. Go to a computer imaging business and have a picture made of yourself in a slimmer body. Put these pictures up where you can see them, and continue to see yourself active and slimmer.

I used to keep a picture of a "slimmer me" on my refrigerator. When I would get upset, angry, or disappointed and race to the refrigerator for a quick fix (HaagenDaz ice cream of course), that picture stopped me! When I looked at that picture, I realized my desire to be thin was greater than my desire to eat ice cream. In fact, that's how I stopped eating ice cream!

So get that picture out again, and remember how good it felt to be thin. Keep it around. Remember that expression, "out of sight, out of mind." If you don't keep seeing your picture, you will forget it. So find whatever works for you. Find some kind of image you can relate to and use it to keep yourself motivated, moving towards your goals.

2. Go Step-By-Step

You may feel overwhelmed if you want to lose a lot of weight, or have never really exercised. Don't focus on the big part. Break it down into many small parts, and take one thing at a time. Can you just walk for 15 minutes a day? Walk around the block, and increase it a little bit at a time. You can do that. Just like you've done anything else in your life. This program allows you to begin with small steps and work your way up.

Last year, I moved into my first home after renting apartments for many years. Well, when you move, you find out what kind of stuff you have been collecting for years. I ran out of time to go through each box before I moved, so I dragged them all with me to the new home and put them in a closet. Thank God for great friends, Luann, Kevin, Veronica, Anne, Wayne, Kyle, and Bill who graciously helped me move all of those boxes upstairs!

Well, it had to happen sometime. I was working on my cookbook, and couldn't find some important papers from classes I had taught. So I decided to look through the boxes. I hadn't even looked at these boxes for years. I just kept collecting more stuff. I guess I figured that the job would be overwhelming. It would take too long to go through all those papers. I saw that project kind of like emptying a swimming pool with a spoon; it would take forever! Well, I needed those recipes, so I decided to look through the boxes, one box at a time. But there were 14 boxes! Night after night, I emptied everything out of each box, one box at a time, one night at a time. It took several weeks before I found those important papers.

Did I have time to sort all those papers? No, but I had to make the time. I found all kinds of things I was looking for, or needed. It took years for me to collect all those papers. It took several weeks for me to go through them and decide what to do with them.

Sometimes we do this with projects like losing weight. We keep letting 10, 20 or 50 pounds accumulate. We wait a year, 2 years, and even 5 years. Finally we decide to change our diet. Well, just like me sorting all those boxes, it's going to take some time to lose weight. We can't be overwhelmed by the first box, and we can't be overwhelmed by the first steps to change.

Let's say you want to change your diet, and your first goal is to eliminate the foods you crave. Sometimes I start people with handling sugar cravings. Or maybe you want to eat more vegetables or salads. Great, make that change. Start somewhere. Anywhere. The more you learn, the more you want to learn. Move a step higher each time. Continue to challenge yourself. Get started and keep going, one step, one box or one pound at a time.

Make new habits and build on them, one at a time. Take the first step. Get moving. Decide, and go forward. Do it one step at a time.

3. Forget the Past

You can't look at two places at the same time. Focusing on your picture or image for fitness helps you not to focus on the past. So if you want to compare, compare yourself with how you will look in the future, not with how you have looked in the past.

After I graduated from high school, I went to a two-year community college in Buffalo. Then I got married and moved to Schweinfurt, West Germany which interrupted my educational plans. But I found classes at the University of Maryland. We kept moving around, and when we returned to the states, we moved to Washington state. I took more night classes, trying to work on my last two years of college. Year after year, I would take as many classes as I could. Finally, many years later, I decided to finish my college degree. But how would I finish it? I would be so much older by the time I would get this degree. The thing was, I would be older no matter if I went back to school or not. I only had one year left, so I went back to school and finally finished a BA in communications at age 34. So what if I didn't just start college and finish like my two sisters? By now they both had their Masters degrees. So what if it took me longer? So what if I was in my mid-thirties when I finally finished? By that age, I had traveled all over the world, and I was a much better student. You're far more focused in your 30s than in your 20s! I'm so glad that I didn't keep focusing on what I hadn't achieved, or how long it took me to finish my BA, but rather the future, and where I was headed.

A few years ago, I lived with a precious Christian woman for nearly three years. We had a great friendship. But I noticed that she saw herself differently than I saw myself. She used to identify herself by what she didn't have—once she told me, "We are both husbandless, and childless." I never saw myself in those terms. So what if I didn't have a husband? So what if I didn't have children? The opportunity was not there for me to have children or a husband. I spent many years giving myself to studying nutrition, motivation, fitness, and later the Bible. None of that time was wasted. We can only do so much. My books were my "babies" and my prayer is that they will be a blessing to my readers.

Never mind the past! Never mind if you've tried to exercise regularly and gave up. Never mind if you have tried to diet and failed every time. Keep working your plan in spite of the past. You're in the Life Cycle now. It's a new day, a new month, a new year. It's time for a new beginning.

Forget the past—it's a new day! Keep your eyes on your goal and don't turn your back.

4. Get Off Your "I Can'ts"

Do you just find yourself sometimes thinking about your "I can'ts?" Do you think about the things you can't do—like exercise and eating better? Then turn your "I can'ts" around. Think about what you can do. Maybe you can't run or roller blade, but you probably can walk. Maybe you're not a gourmet chef, but anyone can make a nice salad.

You can have in life what you focus on. Why focus on what you can't do? Choose what you think about, and what you can do.

Don't allow yourself to make excuses for not changing. How do you get off your "I can'ts?" Change your thoughts and change yourself. Write them down and change them, one at a time. See yourself active, thin, and successful. See it, say it, write it and have it!

When I first started to change my thoughts, I used a journal like I taught you in chapters 4-6. I remember writing things like, "So what if that happened in the past? The past is over. I'm different now. I'm a new person. I can lose weight. I can stick with it. I can succeed and I expect to win."

Remember why you are changing. Begin to say that you can succeed, you can lose weight and you can exercise. The more you keep saying that you can change, the more you believe in yourself. That's developing your faith. Expect more. Expect to change, which really is hope. You probably have that one dress or pair of pants that you bought on sale, just in case you lost weight some day! Grab the faith or hope that you do have and build on that. You have incredible potential inside of you. Stay focused on your goals. Push through those excuses. Pursue your goals with determination and commitment. Keep saying what you want, not what you don't want. Focus on the good things that you are doing. Give it some time. You can override every old image, every old thought. You can become different in your own eyes. You can achieve such great things!

Use Chapters 4, 5 or 6 to help you become aware of what you are saying about yourself, your thoughts about food and exercise and your ability to change.

5. Get Supportive Friends

Try to find supportive encouraging, friends who are not intimidated by your desire for success.

My Pastor, Eastman Curtis is a great example of an overcomer. Kicked out of three schools for drugs and alcohol, he felt like a failure. But one day he met the Lord Jesus Christ, and he was supernaturally delivered from drugs and alcohol. His dramatic conversion and radical transformation caused a revival to explode in his high school campus. He became a leader in his school. He began to get great grades. He went from a flunky to an honor student and Senior Class President. He later went to Bible School, and met his beautiful wife, Angel. They pastor a growing church called Destiny, in Broken Arrow, Oklahoma and have two children.

After 15 years on the road as a traveling evangelist, Pastor Eastman had a dream to produce videos for teens. After he produced his first video, a pastor told him, "You better stay away from TV. It's not your gift. It will get you sidetracked."

Eastman could have let this pastor's comments discourage him. But he remembered his dream, his vision. He thought, *This dream is from God, and He will bring it to pass.* Now his TV show, "This Generation" is rated the number one teen show in America! Don't listen to the discouraging words of other people.

Perhaps You Can!

The first few times I lifted weights, I felt weak and intimidated. I was not able to lift much. One of the trainers kept telling me I could do it. He encouraged me to try harder and push myself. I thought, *If he thinks I can do it, then perhaps I can.* I began to work harder at it and eventually I was able to benchpress *fifty pounds*!

We all need people who believe in us. I'm blessed to have many encouragers—my mother, my sisters, and many friends. When I feel down or discouraged, I call those encouragers to help me regain my perspective. They have helped me turn my focus off my problems and back to working solutions!

After working with an editor on an early manuscript, she basically told me I wasn't a good writer and shouldn't be published! Her feedback discouraged me so much that I couldn't write for about 3-4 months. With the support of great friends, I picked up the pen and finally got published.

Remember the story about Jim Stovall and the four-year old boy named Christopher who encouraged him? One young boy told Jim, "Yes, you can!" Jim's life was changed that day. By now, hundreds of thousands of people have been impacted positively by that story. Find supportive, encouraging friends.

How many times have we held ourselves back because someone told us we couldn't do something? Don't let anyone hold you back from your dreams, goals and purpose. Never mind the negative words that may have been said about you or your potential. Find encouragers and be an encourager. Get a supportive friend and listen to their encouraging words.

6. Get a Success Notebook

Here's another tool that I used a lot in the beginning of my health and weight-loss plan. Celebrate small victories along the way. Plan something special at the end of an allotted period—say at the end of a 7, 14, or 30-day plan. For example, you may buy yourself a new outfit, or a book, or a music tape. Periodically get rid of the clothes that are too big for you and make room for new clothes in your new size. This re-establishes the reality of your weight loss and helps you hold the ground you've taken.

Jot down all of your successes. Even the small ones. Hey, you didn't eat dessert all week? Great! You walked a mile several times this week? Terrific! You didn't drink soda? Wonderful! See your successes on paper.

Why is this important? When you get depressed, do you remember the good things that you have accomplished? No! At that point, all you can see is the food you shouldn't have eaten, or the exercise you didn't do.

If you have a written record of the victories, that record will inspire you and give you hope that things are changing!

So write down what you overcame and when you overcame. You refused to eat donuts on your morning break. You made a healthy lunch every day for an entire week. You never ate late at night for four night in a row. Congratulations!

1. _____
2. _____
3. _____
4. _____
5. _____
6. _____
7. _____
8. _____
9. _____

The more you do healthy things, the more you *want* to do them. Success breeds success. When you are feeling discouraged, get out your *success notebook* and read it out loud to yourself. Remind yourself that you already did it, and you can and will continue to do it!

7. Never Give Up

The one common denominator found among successful people is that they refuse to give up! They keep the picture before them and work toward their goals. If they slip and fall, they get up and start over.

You may fail. Like a boxer, you may get a black eye. You may be knocked to the mat. You may be woozy and not want to get back up (Sounds like the first day on a fad diet!), but the people who know how to win know that as long as they get up again and keep trying, they *will* succeed. The most natural thing to do after getting knocked down is to get back up again. Who wants to just lie there? There's no place to go but up! So come on, get up again! Start over.

Where Else Is There To Go But Up?

Awhile ago, I heard an amazing story about an incredible victory. Gary Davis fell 130 feet out of a drilling rig—and lived to tell about it. Imagine falling off a 13-story building! So many parts of his body were broken: his right arm was broken, his left leg was fractured in eleven places, and his left ankle was shattered. If that wasn't enough, he broke his shoulder blade in five places, broke his collarbone, and all ribs on the left side. His spleen and tailbone were torn out. Gary explained that he had twenty surgeries before he was put together again. But there's more.

Gary had been what they call a roughneck in the oilfield for years. So he never pursued any educational goals. He never thought of himself as being very smart. But while he was recovering, he decided to go back to school to Oklahoma State University and get a degree in Occupational and Environmental Safety. To his surprise, he earned a 4.0 grade point average! Now he wants to learn to be a professional speaker.

I asked Gary what kept him going? How did he stay encouraged? His reply was, "I always had a will to live. I've always strived to be the best at anything I did. Not making it wasn't an option. Where else is there to go but up?"

Just Get Started

The hardest part is often getting started. Once you get going, don't stop. Keep your momentum. Give it everything you've got. Remember all the reasons why you want to change. Don't even consider that you won't succeed. Eventually, you will make new associations, new brain patterns, and new habits. Continually remind yourself of why you wanted to change. Why you want to eat better.

Get back in the groove; get those tennis shoes back on and start moving again. Start eating better. Keep reminding yourself of your goals. Keep doing it long enough to make it a great habit. Remind yourself that you didn't put the weight on overnight, so you won't lose it overnight. But you will lose it if you keep on going. You'll get that motivation back. Your motivation comes with action, as you build it into your life.

Use every tool in this program to help you stay motivated, especially your words. Below are many motivational phrases that I have used to keep myself motivated. Find some that move you to action and keep them before you to never give up!

Keep on keeping on.

You can do it!

Make up your mind and go for it!

Give it everything you've got!

Do more than you've ever done.

Go the extra mile.

Beat the odds.

Take the first step.

Get going and don't stop.

Don't quit!

Keep your eyes on your goal.

Aim high.

Dream big.

See the possibilities.

Do what it takes to win.

You're gonna make it!

Stay focused.

Be persistent.

Make it happen!

It is possible.

There's no excuse for failure.

Face your fears.

Expect to win!

Believe in yourself!

Push yourself.

It's too soon to give up!

Get out of your comfort zone.

See it, say it, write it, have it!

It's never too late.

No one can stop you.

Just do it!

Try harder.

Never give up!

Go beyond what you have done.

Chapter Summary

- How Can You Stay Motivated?
    1. Keep your picture before you.
    2. Go step-by-step.
    3. Forget the past.
    4. Get rid of your "I can'ts."
    5. Get supportive friends.
    6. Get a success notebook.
    7. Never give up.

Motivational Statements:

I can change, one step at a time. I keep my eyes on my goals, and I don't look back. I forget the past, it's a new day. I never give up because I have perserverance. To stay on track, I use my endurance.

STEP FOUR

Plan Your Life

Chapter Nine

How to Really Set Goals

Prior to learning about goal setting, I made the same New Year's resolutions every year: get rid of those extra pounds by starting a diet and exercise program. And every year the same thing happened. I started on a diet around the first week of January. I began taking an aerobics class at the health club, and I even had to fight for a good parking space at 6:00 in the morning. I had to sign-up to get to use the stair stepping machine. But come mid-March, there were plenty of parking spaces and there was no longer a waiting list for the machines. As with dozens of others, my plans were forgotten, along with my thin waist.

And there were times I set goals, but I often became discouraged, like when I did sit-ups faithfully for four months on my living-room floor and the only thing I did was wear out the rug!

Without goals or a clear vision, my efforts were like using the stair-climbing machine—I was expending a lot of energy but going nowhere. But I eventually got results, and you can too.

Perhaps that has happened to you. Your intentions were good. You truly wanted to lose weight, but you lacked the skills of setting goals and carrying through with the plans to make them happen. Understanding how to plan for change in your life is the fourth part of your foundation for change.

It's Natural To Set Goals

Think about what you did today. Did you shop? Run errands? Write a paper? Make a sale? Read a book? Clean the house? Whatever you accomplished was a desired outcome, or a *goal*. You made a mental or written plan and followed through with your plans. It's natural.

You may say, "But those were easy goals to attain. My problem is in setting and accomplishing *harder* goals like losing weight." You can do almost anything if you just break it down into small enough parts, and work on them one part at a time.

I started setting goals for my body and weight. Whoever said, "Inch by inch, anything's a cinch," didn't know that each *inch* could take months! Sometimes it seemed so long before I saw results that my "eyes of faith" needed bifocals. But I pressed on and through faith and patience I have received my reward of thin thighs and a tiny waist!

Why Set Goals?

1. To Get Focused

Prior to setting specific goals, I felt lazy, scattered, and unmotivated. I had no major plan to direct my life or my efforts to lose weight. I would attend aerobics classes for a time, then drop out after a few months. Then I'd see an advertisement for a dance-type class which excited me. I'd sign up and attend for a time, and then drop out.

But when I set definite weight-loss goals, and developed a plan for achieving them, I became focused. I saw all the parts involved on paper and it seemed more possible. The more you can see that something is possible, the more you will try to attain it.

Once I became focused with goal setting, I wasn't enticed into trying every new thing that came along. I no longer wasted time on unproductive activities. My life became more directed, and more exciting.

Sometimes as you set goals, you'll see more parts to the plan as well. I remember hearing a funny story years ago by a teacher named Wyatt Brown. He was talking about trying to get money to plan a trip to a Six Flags theme park. He was concerned as he was budgeting money for gas, the hotel, and the theme park. He turned to his wife, and said, "I suppose you want to eat too?"

Your goals and plans may expand as you work on them!

2. To Keep Your Picture Before You

You get what you focus on. Remember when I told you that I had a picture of a thin me with motivational statements where I could see them? At one time I had so many pictures up and motivational statements posted, that guests in my home wondered if I was trying to lose weight, or start my own health club! But everything helped me move towards my goals.

Seeing my goals written on pieces of paper constantly reminded me of my vision and helped me to stay on track. It kept me focused, motivated, and it kept me from procrastinating.

Think about the time when you were successful at weight loss. Did you set goals? Even in your head? More than likely you did. When you set goals and set a time frame in which to achieve them, your motivation increases. You can imagine that it is possible.

Each time you read your goals list, you start to believe in them. Goals give you a place to begin. Goals can be your "jump start" to weight loss and victory.

3. To Inspire Your Creativity

People can be so creative! I'm amazed at the number of ideas that my clients come up with to help themselves achieve their goals. One client, Gaye didn't like the Food Diary that I was giving to my clients and designed one for herself. I liked it so much that with her permission I started to use her Food Diary with my clients and now in my book. A version of her chart is in chapter 17.

Other clients find creative ways to get more exercise or experiment with new recipes.

Life can become boring, if we let it. We get up, get dressed, go to work, come home, eat, watch television, sleep, and then start all over again. I was bored, depressed, and lacked energy until I found purpose in projects. Now I have a reason to get up every day. I love encouraging people.

In the past, I've challenged myself to be more creative. In the late 70s, I studied calligraphy for three years and dabbled with cartooning. I didn't know that I would be any good at any of these things; I just wanted to try. To my surprise, I was fairly good. About ten years ago, I began studying how to write humor. My first speech in a Toastmasters Regional Contest was a humorous speech. I didn't take first place, but people enjoyed my speech and it made life exciting. Not too long ago, I did a stand-up comedy routine at a New Year's Eve singles party. I still challenge myself to try new things!

It's far more exciting to be creative than to sit around and watch the fruit of others' creativity. Everyone is creative—including you! Where is it? How could you make losing weight fun? What if you asked your family to start exercising with you? Or, what if you made your menu planning a family project? One of your children may be a future gourmet chef!

Beyond weight loss, what do you love to do? What are the things that you've always wanted to try but never have done?

If you are bored with life, decide to aggressively pursue and gain new knowledge and you will find new avenues opening up.

4. To Build Confidence

The more you set goals and really accomplish them, the more confidence you gain. You can't help it! I never knew I could write one book, much less four. The more you do anything, the better you get.

That confidence can carry over into other parts of your life. I've met clients who lost weight, and it changed their lives. They got a new job, or found a spouse. It's always worth the time and effort you put in to change yourself or your life.

Just the process of writing goals helps you imagine that your life can be better. Years ago, I wrote down some goals for a house and new car. For 12 years, I drove an old Volkswagen Fox, year after year, so I could save money for a nice car some day. I had several car accidents within a two year period several years ago, so I wanted a car that was really safe and secure to me. My friend Bill helped me to think about what I really wanted. We went to a few lots, and I really wanted a Volvo but I didn't like the original style. They had just changed the Volvo and I fell in love with the Volvo S40. So I bought it. Of course, after buying a new car, I had to move to a house with a garage. This is like buying a pair of shoes and needing a dress to go with it!

From setting goals earlier, I knew what kind of house I wanted; I knew what I was looking for. I felt impressed by the Lord to look at a townhouse one day, and four months later, I was in that townhouse. The interesting thing was that more than ten years ago, I wrote down goals for a new car and a townhome with some pictures I cut out of a magazine. The picture of the home and car were surprisingly similar to my new townhome and car!

What About You?

Are you setting goals? Why not?

Think someone is holding you back? Maybe, but for most of us we hold ourselves back by our own limited thinking and wrong behavior. No one was forcing me to eat. And no one kept me from exercising. Once I got honest with myself, I saw that no person ever held me back. I was the one responsible for my health and body. People can't hold us back unless we let them.

What if I Make a Mistake?

Maybe you are afraid to make a mistake. Mistakes aren't all bad. Failure to try is much worse than making mistakes. I didn't know if my books would sell when I wrote them. Some things you just don't know until you try! But what if you do succeed? What if you make a positive impact on hundreds or thousands of lives! How exciting!

You'll never know how well you can do something until you try. Mistakes can offer valuable feedback. Everyone fails from time to time; it's quite natural. How does a child learn how to walk? He falls down and gets back up, falls down and gets back up, over and over again. He eventually learns to walk. We are the same way.

Everyone knows how Edison discovered 1,000 ways *not* to make the light bulb before he got it right. Learn from your mistakes and the mistakes of others. Through this book, hopefully you will learn from *my* mistakes! Successful people win in spite of their mistakes and you can too.

Or, maybe you just don't know how to put goals in your life. There was a time when I had no idea how to plan. I'd start things and quit, over and over until I learned how to use the Life Design Planning Chart featured in the next chapter.

This chart helped me to integrate my goals into my life on a daily basis.

Steps for Setting Goals

1. Set Realistic Goals

In every weight loss class I teach, there is at least one person who insists on losing weight faster than the recommended ½ - 1 pound a week. They've tried so many quick weight loss plans, they're geared to thinking "Do it fast." But *quick* weight loss is the least successful way to lose weight permanently.

Slower is better because you are not losing *weight*, you are losing *fat*. Trial and error teaches us how to be more realistic. When people make their goals so unrealistic they can't possibly achieve them, they're defeated before they begin. It's not wise to try to lose fifty pounds more quickly than you put them on. By following the steps in this section, you will be able to set reasonable, achievable goals.

Even though your main goal is weight loss, you'll need goals in other specific areas—walking every day or cutting down on sugar. We'll be changing a lot of behaviors—so why not be specific with some of these behaviors? Weight loss will be easier and more permanent.

Other unrealistic goals are things we say to ourselves, such as, "I'm going to exercise every day for one hour." Set exercise goals of 15-20 minutes every other day and build from there.

Base your current goals on your current time allotments and physical abilities. Let's take exercise as an example. You may choose to walk or do aerobics five times a week. Most people can plan exercise on the weekends so that accounts for two days. Finding an additional three to four more days to exercise might be hard, but finding one or two days might not be. So exercising twice on the weekend and twice in the week might be a realistic goal; anything over that might be unrealistic.

Pay attention to your physical abilities. If your exercise program now consists of letting your "fingers do the walking" through the Yellow Pages, you might want to begin with a walking program as opposed to a strenuous jogging program.

2. Write Them Down

Get them on paper, and with a deadline. If you know what you want to accomplish by a certain date, you can know what you will have to do each day to get there. Writing down your plan and your steps to achieve the plan helps you identify what you want, when you want it, and how to get it. Again, this motivates you when you see it on paper because you can begin to imagine in your mind that it is possible.

What exactly do you want? How many pounds do you want to lose? What size dress (or slacks) do you want to wear? What exercises will you do? When? Where? By what date? The more specific you are with your goal lists, the more likely you will succeed.

How many times have you and a friend said, "Hey, let's do lunch sometime." And how many times have you really had lunch together? Unless you have a definite date, it may be forgotten. We aim towards targets, and without one, we lose our motivation. Set some kind of target date to keep you moving forward.

3. Set Many Small Goals

I used to feel overwhelmed by big goals. Then I learned how to divide my goals into what I like to call "sub" goals. It was easier to imagine losing five pounds than forty. It was easier to cut down on one or two foods than to think I had to throw away all the food in my kitchen.

Break down your entire plan into smaller pieces. You achieve more when you work consistently. The smaller the parts you identify, the more manageable they will be and the more motivated you will be to change.

Taking small steps applies to every area of your life. The thought of writing a book was once out of the realm of my imagination. So I started with a smaller goal—a chapter at a time or fifteen minutes a day. By taking smaller steps, I finished the book. Now I can work on a book for 8 hours a day. After I broke it down into manageable steps, the work of writing suddenly became fun.

Try setting your weight goals in three stages, depending on how much you want to lose. For example, when I weighed 150, I decided to get down to 140 and stabilize there. Then I got down to 130 and did the same thing. From there, I got down to between 112 and 115. The overall weight loss was about 35 pounds but it seemed more manageable when I broke it down into smaller goals. I couldn't picture myself at 115 when I weighed 150, but I could picture myself at 130. I re-adjusted my image as I achieved success.

You may lose at a different rate than I did. The key is to understand yourself and your lifestyle, and the basics of change, so you can stay at that weight after you lose. Setting short term goals gives you the encouragement and motivation needed to continue your progress. It's easier to lose five pounds than it is thirty. When you lose the first four or five pounds, then you'll be ready for the next goal.

The same short, medium, and long-term goal plan works for changing eating habits as well. Start small and work up. You may start by eliminating sweets, then add more salads and vegetables. Finally, you're making gourmet, tasty, healthy meals!

4. Track Your Success

If you want to lose weight, plan it in increments, rather than just a general number of pounds with no boundaries. Weighing on a scale isn't the most accurate form of measurement, because muscle weighs more than fat.

I recommend you continue to keep track of your measurements: bust, waist, hips and thighs. (Men will keep track of measurements for chest, waist and hips.) Or, just find a piece of clothing or a belt that you want to wear and pay attention to how loose your clothes are.

Set Short, Medium, and Long-Term Goals

Below are weight and exercise goals so that you can design them for the rest of your life. Fill in each of the blanks:

1. My current weight_____ Date _____

2. What is the best weight for my body for the rest of my life? _____ (long-term goal)

3. My short-term goal is _____ by _____

4. My mid-way goal is _____ by _____

5. I want to lose a total of _____ pounds

6. I want to lose _____ pounds a week. (We recommend that you do not exceed 2 pounds per week; ½ to 1 pound a week is safest)

I want to wear a _____ size dress

Or _____ size slacks

(the best size for my metabolism, lifestyle and body frame)

8. I want to exercise by doing _____, _____times a week for _____minutes.

Since successful weight loss involves eating the right kinds of foods at the right time, in the right amounts and exercising regularly, that's where you want to set sub goals. Check the ones you want to work with. I've added blank lines so you can add your own.

Setting Goals in the Six Areas

1. Get a Good Foundation for Change

_____ I want to get in the positive life cycle concerning my weight

_____ I want to make better use of my time

_____ I want to understand my own habits

_____ I want to learn how to set goals

_____ I want to get a vision of myself as the way I want to be

_____ I want to plan my diet better

_____ I want to plan my exercise better

_____ I want to understand change better

_____ _____

_____ _____

_____ _____

2. Think About the Right Things

_____ I want to understand my thinking

_____ I want to renew my mind in areas that are holding me back

_____ I want to change my self-image

_____ I want to change my body image

_____ I want to control my emotions

_____ I want to be more positive

_____ _____

_____ _____

_____ _____

3. Eat the Right Food

_____ I want to eat the right foods for my body

_____ I want to eliminate coffee/sugar/junk food

_____ I want to eliminate sodas

_____ I want to eliminate too many fats

_____ I want to add more fruits and vegetables to my diet

_____ I want to learn how to cook more healthy meals

_____ I want to feed my family better

_____ I want to get off junk food

_____ I want to eat more chicken and fish

_____ I want to learn how to cleanse my body

_____ _____

_____ _____

_____ _____

4. Start Exercising

_____ I want to start an exercise program

_____ I want to establish a program and stick with it

_____ I want to meet people with whom I can exercise

_____ _____

_____ _____

_____ _____

5. Eat at the Right Time

_____ I want to eat only when my body is really hungry, not to
fill emotional needs

_____ I want to be aware of my body's natural signals for
hunger and full

_____ I want to stop the habit of eating at night

_____ I want to be aware of social triggers for eating

_____ I want to be aware of environmental triggers

_____ I want to be aware of activities that cause me to want to eat

_____ _____

_____ _____

_____ _____

6. Eat the Right Amount

_____ I want to eat only what is sufficient for me

_____ I want to resist temptation when I see it coming

_____ I want to become more aware of the temptation to overeat

_____ _____

_____ _____

_____ _____

Although you may have found a number of areas that
need work, it will be too overwhelming to change everything
at once. Go back over the lists and choose two areas out of the
six that you'd like to work on first. Take a few moments and
write out those two areas and the date when you made the
decision to begin changing. Then write out how you will
accomplish them.

For example, you may want to lose ten pounds in ten
weeks by eating less, eliminating sugar, and walking briskly
for twenty minutes three times a week.

My most important goals for each step are:

1. Good Foundation:_____

2. Right Thoughts:_____

3. Right Food:_____

4. Right Exercise:_____

5. Right Amount:_____

6. Right Time:_____

It's time to put your plan into action. Think about practical steps you will need to take and write them in. (Later, we'll use the Life Design Planning Chart to help you integrate these into your life.)

On the next few pages you will find examples given to get you started. Following my examples, you will find your own goal-setting worksheets that you can copy and use.

Goal Setting Worksheets

l. Goal: Spend time looking at my current behavior and beliefs

What: Use my resources to understand my thinking/behavior

How: Use a pen and notebook

Where: Sit at my desk

When: Every morning between 7-7:15

What could keep me from doing this?
Fear, distractions, procrastination

How will I overcome distractions?

Realize it's more important for me to do it. I will gain more confidence and I will feel better if I *do* it than if I stay in my present condition. If I don't do anything, I will never change!

2. Goal: Change how I think about exercise

What: Figure out my limiting thoughts about exercise

How: Use a journal

Where: In bed

When: Before I go to sleep

What could keep me from doing this?
Lack of knowledge of how to do it.

How will I overcome distractions?

Get started and make it a habit

3. Goal: Eat better food

What: Inventory my kitchen. When I go shopping I will buy more fruits and vegetables and less or no junk food. I'll start to weed out foods I don't want to eat any more. (If you don't want to throw away your convenience foods, donate them to someone you know needs some food.)

How: Physically go to the kitchen and assess what's in there!

Where: In the kitchen

When: Tomorrow or this weekend

What could keep me from doing this?

Conflicting beliefs that I still don't want to change, or it's not worth the effort, or it won't make a difference.

How will I overcome distractions?

I'll spend time writing in my journal to identify, think about and change those limiting thoughts.

4. Goal: Exercise regularly

What: Walk three times a week for 15-20 minutes.

How: Plan to walk around the park or in the neighborhood

Where: Walk in the neighborhood during the week, and the park on weekends

When: Try to go either after work or later in the evening

What could keep me from doing this?

Distractions, phone calls, laziness

How will I overcome distractions?

Write it in my day timer and let my friends and family know my objectives, and even invite them to come with me.

5. Goal: Eat smaller amounts

What: For one week, I will observe what I eat. That's the first step to change. Until I actually observe and record what I'm doing, I won't realize how much I overeat. By using the Food Diary, I will notice how often I overeat and then learn why.

How: I'll use my journal and record when I overeat.

Where: In bed

When: At night, before I go to sleep

What could keep me from doing this?

Not wanting to look at my eating patterns.

How will I overcome distractions?

I'll commit to a decision

6. Goal: Eat when I'm really hungry

What: Become aware of how often I eat by using my Food Diary faithfully (See chapter 17).

How: Write down all the foods I eat or things I drink for a whole week.

Where: At my desk or at the kitchen table

When: Every evening before bed

What could keep me from doing this?

Again, distractions, or not wanting to admit I eat at the wrong time, or admit that I don't even *want* to change.

How will I overcome distractions?

Again, I will have to decide to do this, and then make it a priority to sit down and fill out my eating journal. If I don't, I need to figure out why I'm not doing it. What am I really afraid of?

Goal Setting Worksheets

These worksheets are designed for your own personal use. Copy them and use them as you learn the goal-setting process.

l. Goal:

What:

How:

Where:

When:

What could keep me from doing this?

How will I overcome distractions?

2. Goal:

What:

How:

Where:

When:

What could keep me from doing this?

How will I overcome distractions?

3. Goal:

What:

How:

Where:

When:

What could keep me from doing this?

How will I overcome distractions?

4. Goal:

What:

How:

Where:

When:

What could keep me from doing this?

How will I overcome distractions?

5. Goal:

What:

How:

Where:

When:

What could keep me from doing this?

How will I overcome distractions?

6. Goal:

What:

How:

Where:

When:

What could keep me from doing this?

How will I overcome distractions?

This chapter has focused primarily on goal-setting skills. In the next chapter, you will use this knowledge you have gained and learn how to incorporate your goals into your life by understanding time management and using what I call the Life Design Planning Chart.

Chapter Summary

- Why Set Goals?
    1. To get focused.
    2. To keep your picture before you.
    3. To inspire your creativity.
    4. To build confidence.
- Steps for Setting Goals.
    1. Set realistic goals.
    2. Write them down.
    3. Set many small goals.
    4. Track your success.

Motivational Statement:

It's easy for me to reach my goals when I take it one step at a time.

Chapter Ten

How To Manage Your Time

Have you ever met someone who is so organized and such a great time manager that you are tempted to ask their parents if as babies, did they use a Day Timer, penciling in their diaper changes and later, their baseball games and piano lessons? My friend, Jeff Magee, is like that. He's president of his own company, is a business management consultant and also a professional speaker. He's great at using his time managing tools, and he's extremely effective and lives a balanced life. But he's also generous in sharing his tips and ideas with me and others.

I've known people who were so organized with their time that they had their wedding thank-you notes mailed the day they returned from their honeymoon in Hawaii, their Christmas cards in the mail the day after Thanksgiving, and they file their income tax return two months before the April 15th deadline!

However, this isn't the case for most of us. I've received wedding thank-you notes even six months after a wedding, and Christmas cards after Christmas! And who ever files their income taxes before the deadline? Look at the long lines at the post office on April 15th.

When I finally became convinced that I needed a regular exercise program, my thought was: *I just don't have the time.* My days were already so full, I was looking for activities to *eliminate*, not new ones to add in. And yet, I had no idea where my time went, nor did I know exactly how I was using my time.

People often feel overwhelmed when it comes to finding time to start new projects. But the problem may not always be due to lack of time, the problem may be a lack of time management. Everyone gets the same twenty-four hours a day. Why is it then, that some people can accomplish so much in a day, and others waste the hours and seem to get nothing done?

I used to be one of those who wasted time. But through the years, I studied time management. While writing the first draft of this book, I worked full-time, taught a weight-loss class at a local junior college, and was active in my writer's club and at church. In addition, I worked out regularly, and read and studied one to two hours daily, and still had time to spend with friends. Whew! My only secret was great time management.

We can do so much with time: we can spend time, make time, pass time, fill time, kill time, and find time. Today we have more modern appliances than ever which help us to save time. In spite of that fact, people race around at a frantic pace and are busier than ever. Why? They've added more activities to fill in the hours saved by the time-saving devices!

One of the biggest reasons why people don't exercise and eat better is because they don't know how to *make* the time.

You don't need a stopwatch to be an effective time manager. Managing your time simply means several things. How much time do you have? How much time do you waste? What do you want to do and how long will that take? But again, you gotta wanna! If you are not really motivated to change, then the best time management system in the world will not help!

Let's assume you have 1) identified the areas you want to change, 2) you know where you are now, and 3) you want to—I mean really want to—change!

What Are You Doing?

In order to make time in your schedule for exercise and healthy eating, you have to know what you're doing. By using the time log or a simple calendar to help you, begin to keep track of how you spend each day. (See sample Time Log at the end of this chapter.)

Get a pen and begin by blocking out the hours you work and sleep. For most people those hours will be something like from 8 a.m. to 5 p.m. for work, and from 10 p.m. or 11 p.m. to 6 a.m. or 7 a.m. for sleep.

After these are blocked out, identify your lunch hour and commuting time next. These times slots will remain fairly consistent.

If you want, block out some time for some peace and quiet—or time to reflect on your day or life. Now go back and include other variables like cooking, cleaning, eating meals, grooming, entertainment, running errands, doing housework, studying, and so on.

Once you have filled in your chart, look at it. Where do you waste time? Where do other people control your time? How many hours do you spend working towards your goal of being healthy? Don't be discouraged if you don't see a lot of free time, especially if you work full-time. The idea is to take advantage of the free time you do have, or can make available.

Since time management boils down to priorities, just putting your schedule on paper helps you determine what's most important.

One note about watching television—if you are spending more than ten hours a week watching sitcoms, game shows, and movies that do not edify, then get excited because you have just "found" a treasure chest of time! What is really important? Are any of these things as important as your weight loss and health? You don't have to do anything radical like throw away your television set. Just find some balance.

Send in the Time Cops

Here are suggestions when you might want to send the "time cops" in to recover lost time: What about the time you waste by eating late at night or when you're really not hungry? What about the "lost" time while waiting for a friend to come over? Or waiting for an appointment? A half hour before the news, or before bed?

The more aware you become of how you spend time, the better you'll become at managing time.

Where Do You Need Time?

Do you need time to fix healthy meals, or to start your exercise program? In my weight-loss classes, we often do a "time search" exercise in which the students search for pockets of time to do some of the items in the list below. We begin by allotting a realistic amount of time for each activity and then accounting for it. These activities do take time, so the more we plan for them, the more likely we are to do them. These times will, of course, vary from family to family. In planning for these activities, we just use a simple calendar. Here are several ideas that my students came up with:

1. Plan meals (1/2 hour weekly).
2. Shop for groceries (2-4 hours weekly).
3. Prepare meals (breakfast, lunch, dinner) 2-3 hours daily.

4. Eat meals (1/2 hour for breakfast, 1/2 hour for lunch, 1 hour for dinner, daily).

5. Time for exercise (30 minutes, three to five times a week).

6. Quiet time or prayer (15 minutes, daily).

At the beginning of each week, sit down with your calendar and plan your activities. Budget the time that will be needed for each activity and block out that time on your calendar. The more you have to do, the more detailed your list should be. Once you get it on paper, you will be more likely to stick with your schedule.

I like to shop and plan meals once a week, preferably on Saturday or Sunday. I plan the days and times I will exercise, too. That way it's manageable, but there's also room for flexibility in case plans change.

Seeing these activities on your calendar is like seeing a doctor's appointment. Soon, you will feel as committed to your exercise "appointment" as you are to the doctor's appointment!

Tips for Better Time Management

You are specifically seeking out extra time to: 1) eat well (shop, cook, prepare healthy foods), and 2) exercise. You will also want to allow time to do the important workbook exercises in this program—exercises such as goal-setting.

1. Use Your Time Log

Identify the obstacles that keeping you from exercising. Is there a better time for exercise than what you are currently doing? Had you ever thought of eating a quick "brown bag" lunch in fifteen minutes, and then using the rest of your lunch hour for walking? You will be exercising, relieving stress, and getting out in the fresh air all at the same time.

For you, it may work better to use the hour just before dinner. Or after dinner. This may be a "lost" pocket of time that can be re-discovered and put to better use.

2. Learn to Say, "No"

Are you the type of person who says, "Yes" to every activity? Activities that can waste your time? Activities you don't really want to do? If someone asks you for an obligation that would rob your exercise time, tell the truth about your new program and either suggest another time or have the courage to say, "No."

Most people will understand if you are honest, sincere, and direct. At first, your "no" may seem selfish to you, but is it? Your ability to become involved in outside activities, especially those of helping others, will increase as your health and energy increases.

Give yourself permission to do what you need to do first. Remember, you can't please everyone. Slow down, and don't be so quick to say, "Yes" to requests for your time. You can say, "No."

3. Know Your Limitations

Biting off more than you can chew will lead to frustration, overeating, or even quitting. If you only have a half-hour for exercise, use that half-hour and don't feel quilty. Enjoy the time and make the most of it. Give yourself more to do on the weekend. Even a fifteen-minute walk at the mall is better than nothing.

Time management is not easy for everyone. Perhaps you might ask a friend, relative, or co-worker for assistance to help you plan or manage your time better.

But did you ever consider delegating? Do you have to clean your house, shop, or pick up the kids? Can't you ask someone else to do it? Sometimes we can't do everything, and the small price that we pay is worth great dividends in gained time. Besides, someone else can use the extra money.

Time management is a skill just like any other skill in life. The more you practice it, the better you become. It's all a matter of knowing what you need to do, what your priorities are, and how much time is available. Let's end this chapter by checking the areas where you want to dig up more time.

In which of these areas do you need more time? Check the ones that apply:

_____ 1. Plan meals (1/2 hour weekly).

_____ 2. Shop for groceries (2-4 hours weekly).

_____ 3. Prepare meals (breakfast, lunch, dinner) 2-3 hours daily.

_____ 4. Eat meals (1/2 hour for breakfast, 1/2 hour for lunch, 1 hour for dinner, daily).

_____ 5. Time for exercise (30 minutes, three to five times a week).

_____ 6. Quiet time or prayer (15 minutes or more, daily).

Now that we know how much time we have to use and what we want to do in that time, let's move on to incorporating these ideas into our lives.

Chapter Summary

- Time management is a learned skill.
- Identify what keeps you from doing what you want.
- Tips for better time management.
    1. Use your Time Log.
    2. Learn to say, "No."
    3. Know your limitations.
- Use a time log to seek out lost pockets of time.

Motivational Statements:

I have time for important things like exercise and eating right. There is time to stay healthy and lose weight.

Time Log

HOURS/DAY	MON	TUES	WED	THURS	FRI	SAT	SUN
MORNING							
12:00 - 1:00							
1:00 - 2:00							
2:00 - 3:00							
3:00 - 4:00							
4:00 - 5:00							
5:00 - 6:00							
6:00 - 7:00							
7:00 - 8:00							
8:00 - 9:00							
9:00 - 10:00							
10:00 - 11:00							
11:00 - 12:00							
EVENING							
12:00 - 1:00							
1:00 - 2:00							
2:00 - 3:00							
3:00 - 4:00							
4:00 - 5:00							
5:00 - 6:00							
6:00 - 7:00							
7:00 - 8:00							
8:00 - 9:00							
9:00 - 10:00							
10:00 - 11:00							
11:00 - 12:00							

Chapter Eleven

How To Design
Your Life

Kendra is in the midst of her new weight-loss program. She's only been on it for three weeks. Suddenly, she is overwhelmed with all of the life changes that she wants to make: exercise for twenty minutes a day, cut down on coffee, eliminate sugar, drink more water, eat more fruits and vegetables. In a fit of exasperation, Kendra picks up the phone and calls for a take-out pizza!

Only in America can we order food at any time of the day or night and have it delivered! Maybe that's the real reason for our national weight problem!

Life Design Planning Chart

Through the course of reading this book, you may have already decided you want to make changes and you've accepted the challenge to change. You may have set your goals and learned how you are motivated. Perhaps you've decided that yes, this is the right time for change. But now you may be wondering how will you do it. How will you chart your progress from day to day? How will you know if you are achieving those goals?

I've been using what I call a Life Design Planning Chart for more than nineteen years. (See sample chart at the end of this chapter.) Whenever I want to change a certain area in my life, I use this chart. My ex-husband who had a job training handicapped adults used a chart similar to this one, but he revised it for me. I started using it and it changed how I form habits.

It works something like a "to do" list. For example, let's say I wanted to run three times a week or walk daily for fifteen minutes. I write these down on the chart and begin to track my progress for the next month. As I use the chart, it helps me to establish healthy habits and eliminate bad ones, and it helps to establish new brain/mind connections.

I didn't just use it to start an exercise program and lose weight. I even set goals to learn how to write regularly. Since that time, I've written four major manuscripts, many of them have been re-written several times. It all began with one habit of writing 15 minutes a day.

One Month at a Time

One of the reasons why this chart works is because it's set up in a 30-day segment. That's a good time frame in which to change any habit. A month is a minimum. If you can do something for a month, you can establish a new habit. Psychologically, a month is better than two weeks or 21 days, because you can start over again at the beginning of each new month.

Each month you can re-design your life by getting out your Life Design Planning Chart. Perhaps last month you tried attending a scheduled aerobics class. But this month you want to walk and you want to chart that progress. Later you can compare the two months with each other to see which class was more effective. This helps you to be creative and flexible.

How Does It Work?

Until we write things down on paper, they are vague and undefined. The more you can see and understand something on paper, the more understanding you gain. With this chart, you won't have to reinvent the wheel every day. You'll know what you want to do and you won't be so vulnerable to the temptations which may try to pull you in the wrong direction.

Increase Your Motivation

Another good thing about this chart is that it helps you see how well you are doing, and acts as an additional motivator to keep on going. Just as we can think that we ate less than we did, we can fool ourselves the other way, and think that we ate more than we did.

Both types of feedback are valuable. We can learn from our mistakes, but better than that, we can rejoice in the successes! I remember how excited I got when I went through a whole week without overeating or eating white sugar or junk food. In past years when I was struggling with drinking coffee, I was elated to realize one day that it had been seven months since I'd had a cup of coffee and I didn't even miss it. I was making gradual changes and suddenly sugar and coffee were not interesting to me.

And finally, this chart gives you the feedback you need to notice the relationship between what you are doing and the results you desire. Even your mistakes can give valuable direction.

Notice Your Patterns

Do you consistently exercise on the weekends, but not during the week? For example, do you eat more sugar or fat on the weekends or during the week? What about coffee? Cinnamon rolls? It helps to isolate and identify patterns in the way you eat.

The idea is to keep these things you want to change in front of you and daily track how well you do them over a month's time. Then reassess your lifestyle and changes.

However, this chart doesn't guarantee that you are going to change anymore than making a "to do" list guarantees the chores will be finished. A tool is good only if it's used. Just because you have a lawn mower sitting in the garage doesn't mean you'll cut the grass. You have to use it.

Keeping track of your behavior is a major factor in weight control because you need feedback to change. Consider what it takes to learn anything new. You learn what to do and when you make a mistake, you correct it so you can move forward.

How I Use the Life Design Chart

Think specifically about the habits you want to change and the goals you have set earlier. (Turn back to the goal-setting chapter to do this.) Write these goals in the blank chart. For example, there were several behaviors I wanted to establish, so in the beginning, one of my charts might have looked like this:

1. Spend 5-15 min. of quiet time.
2. Use journal to help change my thinking.
3. Drink 6-8 glasses of water daily.
4. Eat fruits and vegetables.
5. Take my food supplements.
6. Get a couple of servings of protein a day.
7. Exercise 20 min. (3-4 times).
8. Eat when only really physically hungry, not due to external triggers.
9. Eat small portions or appropriate portions of food.

This is just a beginning. You may want to use a separate chart for each idea, or even add more activities under each subject. Every chapter and part of this book is interchange-able—don't be afraid to reread it and work in these chapters, according to your needs and goals.

How You Can Use the Life Design Chart

Here are suggestions for best results with keeping track of your behavior:

1. Fill in the Dates

Starting with today's date, fill in the dates for the remainder of the month, or the beginning of the next month, whichever is closest. Use both the number date and the letter of the day of the weeks: M for Monday, T for Tuesday and so on. This will help you to see relationships later. If you just write in 3/16, you may not remember is that was a weekday or the weekend.

2. Start Small

Don't try to change too many things at once. I wrote down 9 just for an example. Think about the things you really could do in one day. Be realistic. Building one or two habits at a time is more effective than trying to do too much and not developing any new habits. But it's good to start with at least one or two dietary and exercise changes right away to get started on your weight-loss goals.

3. Write Clearly

Be sure to write clear enough so that you can read it later.

How To Change Your Behavior

Once you fill in the chart, here's how to use it to change your behavior:

1. Use Your Chart Every Day

Try to do each of the items listed in your chart every day. The best time to fill your chart is at the end of the day. Don't wait too long to fill in the chart—if you do, you'll forget. You may think you did more than you really did, or vice versa. This is a place where honesty is imperative. Resist the temptation to exaggarate the truth, just as you would resist a gooey jelly-filled donut!

2. Check What You Complete

Put a check mark next to the activity on the day you completed it. For example, if you didn't eat sugar, coffee or extra fat, you put a check mark beside that item under that date.

3. Review Weekly

Review your chart at the end of each week, and notice any correlation. For example, did you notice you had more success in resisting temptations on the days that you exercised? Here is where you will look for emotional, physical and circumstantial patterns in your life. Let me show you what I mean.

a. **Time with self:** Did you spend quiet time reflecting on what you are doing? Did you notice any correlation between this and your weight loss or your weight gain?

b. **Emotional:** Can you correlate your weekend eating to something like loneliness and a Friday night binge? Or phone calls or contact with certain people?

c. **Physical:** Especially for women, do you know your body cycles? Do you, for example, tend to lose control one week before your cycle? What other things do you notice? Any cravings?

d. **Circumstantial:** Is there a day or week when you continually overeat or eat too much sugar? For example, do you have control until every Wednesday morning when you have to attend a weekly staff meeting where there is always a tray of donuts?

4. What Does It Mean?

When you look at your patterns, try not to judge yourself. Be persistent in your efforts to change. Take note of what is working and be aware of ways you can help yourself with more motivation to do certain things.

Perhaps it's unrealistic to attempt to exercise for a full thirty minutes at a time. You may want to cut back to fifteen or twenty minutes a day, or try using time on your lunch hour. You could later set a goal to increase that time, but if you make it too hard, it will kill your motivation. It's better to start small and be consistent with fifteen minutes, than to set your goal for an hour and never reach the goal.

5. Slowly Add New Activities

As you progress in your chart and gain confidence and consistency with these activities, you can update your chart by adding new activities you want to incorporate into your routine. Add things that will track your feelings of self worth, or moods, for example. Generally, the more you accomplish something the better you feel about yourself, and this chart will help you to achieve this too.

Most of us are not good at knowing just how we are doing. Whenever we learn something new, we need feedback. The Life Design Planning Chart gives you an excellent source of feedback. At a glance, by looking at your check marks, you can see when you accomplished your goals and when you didn't. This chart also indicates areas in which you are resistant to change. After a month, study your chart and decide if you want to continue doing what you were doing.

Ask yourself key questions. Perhaps you were able to eat better, but weren't consistent in your exercise. Ask yourself why? Was it too hard? Too long? Too inconvenient? Perhaps there is something else that you could try that would fit into your routine better. Begin to list other options.

You have written your behavior goals on this chart and have made a plan to do them. As your new habits become stronger, the old bad ones will become weaker. You will be motivating yourself to not give up. If you remain consistent and don't give up, you will reach your goals. Soon your body will reflect the changes that are in the chart!

Keeping track of the changes you want to make, gives you direction, focus and motivation. You will gain more confidence in your ability to change by using the Life Design Planning

Chart. The records prove that you are changing, which then becomes a history of your success. You will also strengthen your beliefs that you can change, because you are changing. You are getting in and staying in the Life Cycle of Fitness.

Chapter Summary

- Use the Life Design Chart for charting progress.
- Keeping track of changes gives direction, focus and motivation.
- How To Change Your Behavior
  1. Use your chart every day.
  2. Check what you complete.
  3. Review weekly.
  4. What does it mean?
  5. Slowly add new activities.

Motivational Statements:

Planning my life is easy. Making new habits is easy.

Life Design Planning Chart

Name _____ _____ Weight/Size Goal

Activity																										
1																										
2																										
3																										
4																										
5																										
6																										
7																										
8																										
9																										
10																										
11																										
12																										

PART TWO

The Physical Side
of Change

STEP FIVE

God's Healthy Provision

Chapter Twelve

Eat Fat-Burning Foods

Karen is a client who told me that she really wanted to change her diet, but she had to go slowly. For Karen, taking her first step was ordering fat-free French fries to lower the fat in her diet. When she received her order, the fries were dripping with fat. She asked the waitress, "Did you tell me these French fries were fat-free? The waitress replied, "Oh, yes, you pay for the potatoes, the fat is free!" Well, at least it's a start!

In Part One, we talked about the mental side to change. In Part Two, we'll look at the physical side, starting with diet.

Why Am I So Tired?

I can relate to overweight clients who come into the office for the first time and say, "I really want to exercise, but I'm too tired!" Their disappointment is often combined with feelings of guilt like there is something terribly wrong with them. Why can't they "just do it?"

Many years ago, I was a tired, depressed, cranky calorie counter! I wrote my first book, *Why Can't I Lose Weight?* because I had learned about so many physical imbalances that made me tired. In chapter 7, I mentioned these: 1) Fatigue from nutritional deficiencies (like the B complex); 2) Fatigue from hypothyroid (low thyroid) or hypoadrenal (low adrenal); and 3) Lack of knowledge about how your body works. You may be eating foods that are making you tired, fat and depressed.

Uh-oh! It's incredibly hard to be motivated to do anything, much less get the energy to make major lifestyle changes and start an aggressive exercise routine when you are exhausted! It's not a matter of hype or pumping yourself with affirmations or confessions! You can't confess away iron deficiency. Rather, it's a matter of eating foods that give you optimal energy, and working with how your body was designed. So in this chapter we'll get to the bottom line of fat-burning, energy-producing foods.

Read Any Diet Books Lately?

Browsing through your local bookstore, you'll see dozens of books on diets. Some books advocate a high-protein, low-carbohydrate diet; while others tell you to eat a high-carbohydrate, low-protein diet. Still others advocate a high-fiber diet or vegetarian diet. Then there are blood or body type diets. Even if you've only read one or two of these books, you may be confused when the authors start to contradict each other!

I can see as many as 30 follow up-appointments a day, and I've interviewed thousands of people in the last 15 years. I've met people who eat only twice a day and keep their weight normal. I've had clients who eat moderate protein and are healthy and losing weight. I've worked with body builders and vegetarians. I've had a first-hand opportunity to see what is really working and where people have problems. And I've been able to help some people who were at a plateau finally lose those last 10 pounds. When I wrote my first book, I didn't want to add to the confusion; in fact, I wanted to explain it.

What Really Makes Us Fat?

So what does Dr. Robert Atkins' high-protein, low-carbohydrate diet, or Dr. Dean Ornish's high-carbohydrate, low-protein diet and the Diamond's semi-vegetarian (*Fit for Life*) programs have in common? They all encourage you to eliminate the junk foods (candy, cakes, cookies, ice cream, etc.—you know, the stuff we all hate to give up!) and hydrogenated or damaged vegetable oils which are linked to increased free radical damage and cancer growth. Packaged, refined processed foods, sugar and damaged fats are the major factor in our diets that cause the most disease. People can lose weight on all three of these plans by just eliminating the junk.

Have you seen the typical American diet lately? Take a peak at the office break room, and see what's there. What's quick, tasty, and easy to take to the office for a reward? How about a birthday? Or an anniversary? Sweets! Pick from cakes, cookies, donuts, or sweet breads. It's American, it's tradition, and it's settled! We reward ourselves with sweets, usually sweetened with refined white sugar. You know, the "pure" stuff.

Eliminating sugar and white sugar products, processed carbohydrates and processed or bad fats makes sense. Let's look at all three regarding weight loss. Then I'll give you general guidelines for eating to lose weight.

Sugar, the New Kid on the Block

You and I may have grown up eating refined white sugar, but did you know that chemically refined white sugar is fairly recent? According to Mary June Parks in *A New You*, for centuries, sugar was sold by the teaspoonful only through drug stores.[1] Originally crude, unrefined beet sugar was a luxury.

For most of the world's population, for hundreds of thousands of years, people didn't eat sugar. The word "sugar" is not in the Bible, having been used only in the last hundred years. A comparable Bible food was honey, which also needs to be used in moderation (Prov. 25:27: *It is not good to eat much honey*).

These are not real foods, but rather processed foods. Can you imagine Adam and Eve in the garden eating a Twinkie? I still think they preferred apples!

In the late 1970s, *Sugar Blues* by William Duffy made us aware of the possible dangers of a diet high in refined sugar. That book is still in print, and sugar consumption still matters! In the 1800s, the Average American ate about 10 pounds of sugar per year. Today, individual consumption of sugar has skyrocketed, especially with the increase in low-fat or fat-free products. Today the average American consumes 170 pounds of sugar per person per year!

You, Too, Can Increase Your Risk for Diabetes

It's no wonder that diabetes is one of the fastest-growing diseases with more than 2,000 people being diagnosed daily. According to the American Diabetes Association, in the U.S., approximately 16 million people have diabetes. The incidence of diabetes has increased six-fold since 1930, and according to the Center for Disease Control and Prevention, in the past 10 years the incidence of diabetes has increased 75%. The risk for heart disease and stroke increases tremendously when a person has diabetes.

While the sugar industry denies that sugar is hazardous to human health, I'm looking forward to the day that foods will be labeled according to what they do to us. Here's one for sugar: "This is a diabetes-inducing, fat-storing, and disease-producing substance. Eating this food may make you crave sweets, increase your risk of heart disease, and make you fat!"

The U.S. Department of Agriculture says that 10 teaspoons of refined sugar is okay every day, but remember sugar isn't a food; it's a toxic, processed substance. Not only do processed foods contain little if any nutrition, they deplete your store of vital vitamins and minerals. And they are packed with preservatives that our body was not designed to deal with. Dr. Feingold wrote about the link between artificial preservatives and hyperactivity in the 60s and 70s. Do you know how long a Twinkie can last? Some people have speculated for many, many years! George Burns once quipped that he loved junk food; he needed all the preservatives he could get! Unfortunately, we can't preserve ourselves with junk foods.

The average American doesn't just eat 10 teaspoons; they eat more like 20 or more teaspoons per day. That total is the amount of sugar. It doesn't take into consideration the amount of processed carbohydrates like white bread and pasta which turn to sugar in the body.

How Can We Eat That Much Sugar?

Why do we eat so much sugar? Everywhere we turn, we are invited to eat sugar. Dessert trays. Big gulp size sodas. Ice cream sundae commercials. I've seen a commercial whose message is that you're grown up now, so you can eat anything you want. In fact, much advertising makes responsible parents look foolish when they are the only ones who don't want their children eating tons of sugar at the day care center.

Children should not be in charge of their own diet! Invariably when children cry and get their own way and the parents give in, the children are the sickest and unhealthiest. These children grow up with great potential for chronic fatigue, diabetes, allergies, asthma, and heart disease. Loving your children means you care about what they put in their mouths as well as what clothes they wear and what they watch on TV. How we eat as a young person determines our health later in life. Disease doesn't just happen. And you might be surprised at how many diseases are not genetically linked at all. We get what our parents get because we eat like our parents ate.

Sugar is so toxic, that getting a stomach ache after eating sugar is a real, natural response. But we override it by giving our children a little sugar every day, to where our digestive system eventually says, "I give up." Your stomach stops sending obvious messages like nausea or vomiting. Instead, it just gets more and more irritated. Later on, we "develop" symptoms like allergies and autoimmune diseases or leaky gut and digestive problems. I'm amazed how many children and parents have miraculously gotten rid of allergies or skin problems when they just eliminated sugar and processed foods from their diet.

If you are craving sugar, get a Chromium with the Glucose Tolerance Factor (Chromium GTF) and take it regularly. You may also need the B complex. If you have an eating disorder, you desperately need zinc. Clinical research has proven that without zinc, a person's perception of themselves is thrown off. This is why people who are anexoric think they are still fat! If you crave chocolate, start with a magnesium supplement. And if you crave carbohydrates, you'll have to eat less carbohydrates. (For more information on cravings, see my weight loss-book.)

It All Adds Up

My friend and teacher, Dr. Michael Dobbins shows how we can easily get 3 cups of sugar in the average American diet:

Breakfast: Cereal, white toast, orange juice and banana: about 1 cup sugar

Lunch: Yogurt with fruit, baked potato, white bread and chicken: 3/4 cup sugar

Three o'clock snack: candy bar and soda: 1/2 cup sugar

Dinner: Pasta, white bread, soda: 3/4 cup sugar

Three cups of sugar translates to about 24 teaspoons of sugar a day!

But did you realize that one can of soda alone contains between 10 to 14 teaspoons of sugar? And it's easy for the average teenage boy to get 34 teaspoons of sugar, with almost 40% of that coming from soft drinks. As I said earlier, today the average American eats 170 pounds of sugar, per person per year. Sixty to seventy-five percent of the population eats like this! Was this way of eating natural?

The Government's Food Pyramid, which recommends 6-11 servings of carbohydrates can easily provide 250-500 grams of carbohydrates a day. No where in history has man eaten that many carbohydrates. I quoted the authors of *Sugar Busters* in my weight-loss book, who said that we have more stress in one day on our pancreas than our ancestors had in a lifetime![2]

1. How Sugar Makes Us Fat

Eating sugar or refined carbohydrates raises the amount of circulating insulin. Why is this significant? Because insulin is the fat-storing, hunger hormone! Eating protein raises the circulating glucagon, which is the fat-burning, anti-hunger, hormone. Is it any wonder then, that body builders can be leaner than carbohydrate-eating people? Is it any wonder that books like *The Atkins Diet, Stillwell Diet*, and *Protein Power* are selling well?

How unfortunate that we have to go to such extremes for weight loss. I know many people who have followed these diets, and when they stopped them, they gained the weight back even quicker. These diets are unbalanced and they often lack minerals, enzymes, important fiber and essential fat.

2. How Carbohydrates Make Us Fat

Do we have to give up pasta, bread, potatoes? Since the Government's new Food Pyramid, now half the population is overweight. Many people ate a "low-fat" diet that only complicated their weight loss problem because they cut out the fat and ate more sugar and carbohydrates.

Unfortunately, much of the nutritional guidelines we follow are given to us by the food industries that make processed foods, not by clinical nutritionists or scientists.

There are two ways to eat carbohydrates and still lose weight. First, cut down the total number of carbohydrates, and second, eat carbohydrates that are high in fiber, like slow-cooking oatmeal, or real whole grain bread—not the white stuff that has been colored with caramel coloring!

3. How Fats Make Us Fat

Obviously, too much of any fat can make us fat. That's why we all cut out fat. But when we cut fat out of our diets, the unfortunate thing was that we cut *all* fat out. We cut out the *good* fats as well as the bad fats. Bad fats are processed fats. They can put weight on because they are so indigestible. These bad fats include vegetable oils which were damaged in processing with high temperatures or chemicals, and hydrogenated and partially hydrogenated oils, such as margarine and Crisco. In the hydrogenation process, hydrogen molecules are added to a perfectly good vegetable oil which damages the fat and also makes it saturated. These damaged fats are linked to free radical damage, heart disease and cancer. So read labels, throw away margarine, and eliminate all deep-fried foods.

What about all of these hydrogenated fake butters that don't melt and taste awful? Butter is better. Hydrogenation is great for preserving the food, but not for preserving us. If the food you are considering buying starts with the phrase, "I can't believe it's...." you probably can believe that it's not a real food! I can't believe that people still buy these foods!

Good Fats Burn Fat

Going fat-free or no-fat is no fun! Like some of my clients, when I tried to not eat fat, I found myself squeezing Haagen-daz in my otherwise healthy diet. God made us to need and enjoy good fat.

Did you know that adding good fat to your diet can help you burn fat? In my weight loss book, I quoted Udo Urasmus who gave several tablespoons of flaxseed oil to one of his clients and she lost 80 pounds![3] Adding one tablespoon of flaxseed oil to your diet daily can help you burn fat.

Protein Power

We've discussed sugar, carbohydrates, and fats; now let's look at protein. While I don't recommend a high-protein diet, I have found that many of my female clients, in their desire to eat healthy really don't eat enough protein or the good type of fat.

Did you know that approximately 100 years ago, heart attacks were scarce in the US? In the early 1900's only about 3% of us died from heart disease. Today, nearly half of our population has some type of heart disease. Wait a minute. Realize what we were eating in the early 1900's: fresh, whole foods, meat, butter and even lard! So why didn't they all die of heart attacks?[4]

Several factors contribute to this. One, the quality of meat and dairy were better; the animals were healthier and since they ate better food, like us, they didn't need so many antibiotics. More importantly, oils weren't refined yet. Today, there is a great link between heart disease and damaged fats, also called trans fatty acids. Hydrogenated fats (where a vegetable fat is hydrogenated and becomes solid, as in the case of margarine) are a leading cause of heart disease.

Second, the lack of nutrition in our diet, even the prevalent vitamin B complex deficiency is linked to heart disease. The B complex and folic acid are proven to reduce the amount of the toxic amino acid homocysteine, which is linked to heart disease.

And finally, high amounts of sugar and refined foods are linked to heart disease. In their book, *Sugar Busters,* the authors say that dietary sugar is recognized as an independent risk factor for cardiac disease. They say that insulin is the hormone that regulates your blood sugar, but it also causes your body to store excess fat and inhibits the mobilization of previously stored fat. And insulin signals our liver to make cholesterol! They point out that most diabetics who take insulin experience higher cholesterol and triglyceride levels as a side effect.[5] By the way, there is little clinical evidence that dietary cholesterol is the risk factor for raising cholesterol. In short, eating eggs doesn't necessary raise your cholesterol. However, if you eat a high-sugar, high-carbohydrate diet, then no matter what else you eat, you will raise your cholesterol. High cholesterol was not even an issue until the 1970s.

There are clinical studies in the *American Journal of Clinical Nutrition* that clearly show a relationship between what a country eats and the rate and types of diseases. You may have heard about the "French Paradox" where people eat more fat than we do, but aren't as fat as we are. We are the only ones who call it a paradox. They just don't eat as many processed foods as we do. Ever hear about the "Spanish Paradox?" In some parts of Spain, Spaniards eat meat like Americans do, but they eat fruits, vegetables, olives, olive oil and meat. According to research, the good fat protects them from heart disease.

My experience with thousands of people shows that if you were to eat just protein, or a high-protein diet, then if you ever eat many carbohydrates you'll probably gain weight even more quickly than you lost it.

The key to eating protein is to balance it with lots of good fats, fresh fruits and vegetables and small amounts of carbohydrates. Choose the best proteins: lean proteins which are not processed.

Fruits and vegetables are wonderful, rich sources of antioxidants, minerals and enzymes. Limit your fruits to two servings a day, but load up on the vegetables which you can eat freely. A meat, vegetable and fruit diet has proven extremely beneficial for people with allergies, asthma, candida, and other allergy-type diseases.

Put Them Together

A good eating plan would include:

2-3 servings of protein a day

2 fruit servings a day

5 vegetable servings a day

1-3 carbohydrate servings a day

1 tablespoon of flaxseed oil a day

If you aren't losing weight then cut out the evening carbohydrate serving.

Daily Servings

At the end of this chapter, I've made a list of fruits, vegetables, proteins, fats and dairy products. Here is a look at daily servings.

Healthy carbohydrates: 1/2 cup oatmeal, millet, beans, lentils, sweet potatoes, 1 slice whole grain breads and 1/2 cup vegetables such as carrots, corn and potatoes.

Healthy proteins: (3 oz. for women; 6 oz. for men) Salmon, tuna, halibut, eggs, lamb, cheese, soy milk, tofu, and lean red meat (steak, hamburger, venison or buffalo meat.) Processed meats (such as sausage and luncheon meats) contain nitrates and nitrites which are linked to cancer.

Healthy fats: (1 tablespoon) flaxseed oil, extra virgin olive oil, expeller pressed canola oil, 10 raw nuts including almonds, cashews, walnuts and hazelnuts; 1/4 c. seeds such as sesame seeds and sunflower seeds.

Healthy vegetables: (1/2 cup) Broccoli, Brussels sprouts, cabbage, cauliflower, celery, cucumber, greens, eggplant, green beans, onions, mushrooms, Romaine lettuce, tomatoes, and sprouts.

Healthy fruits: (1 piece of fruit, or 1/2 cup) Apples, apricots, berries, banana, cherries, grapefruits, grapes, melons, oranges, papaya, peaches, pears, pineapple, plums, tangerines.

Sample Meals

Breakfast: 1/2 cup oatmeal or 2 eggs or 1/2 cup of cottage cheese or protein drink

Lunch: Protein, vegetable and carbohydrate

Dinner: Protein, vegetable and carbohydrate

Fruits:	**Vegetables:**	
apples	artichokes	mushrooms
dates	asparagus	mustard greens
apricots	beets	onions, red
figs	bok choy	onions, white
grapefruit	broccoli	parsnips
blackberries	brussels sprouts	peas
blueberries	cabbage, red	potatoes, red
boysenberries	cabbage, white	potatoes, sweet

Fruits:

raspberries
strawberries
cherries
grapes
watermelon
honeydew
crenshaw
cantaloupe
nectarines
pineapples
plums
oranges
peaches
pears
papaya
tangerines
bananas
mango

Vegetables:

cabbage, savoy
carrots
cauliflower
celery
celery root
chard
corn
daikon
dandelion greens
eggplant
endive
fennel
garlic
green beans
kale
leeks
lettuce, red leaf
lettuce, green leaf
lettuce, romaine

radishes
rutabega
sea vegetables
shallots
snow peas
spinach
squash, acorn
squash, butternut
squash, hubbard
squash, pumpkin
turnips
watercress
parsley
alfalfa sprouts
bean sprouts
water chestnuts
bamboo shoots

Meats/fish/poultry:

Lean beef
veal
lamb
cornish hens
chicken
turkey
trout
swordfish
salmon
ocean perch
whitefish
tuna
mackerel
red snapper

Grains/Beans:

barley
couscous
kasha
millet
brown rice, long
brown rice, short
brown rice, sweet
corn
oat meal
oat bran
rye
wheat
garbanzos
lentils
green split peas
aduki beans

Dairy:

yogurt
white cheeses
kefir
butter
cottage cheese
eggs

Nuts/seeds:

almonds
walnuts
cashews
sesame seeds
sunflower seeds
pecans
caraway seeds
poppy seeds

Oils: **Grains/Beans:**

olive   black-eyed peas
canola   kidney beans
sesame   great northern beans
safflower   navy beans

Animal Protein Meals

*Chicken salad with greens, curried yogurt dressing

*Low fat cottage cheese with veggies or fruit and whole-grain crackers

*Turkey salad in pita bread with sprouts

*Tuna casserole with steamed broccoli, mixed veggies

*Broccoli quiche with onion soup

*Light vegetable or chicken or fish quiche with green salad

*3 oz. sliced turkey breast, mixed green salad, steamed vegetables

*3 oz. water packed tuna, mixed greens with lemon/oil dressing

*Baked fish with lemon and herbs, steamed cauliflower or spinach, salad

*Tuna and vegetable salad with optional steamed squash

*Sliced chicken, sliced tomato with basil dressing and steamed vegetables

*Grilled salmon with steamed asparagus and lemon, sliced cucumbers and tomato

*Sliced turkey with cucumber, tomato, radish salad and steamed broccoli

*Broccoli, carrot and chicken or turkey stir fry with steamed green beans

*Oven baked chicken breasts and steamed onions, peas and greens with carrot/cucumber salad with dressing

*Tuna, salmon, beef, or chicken with tossed green salad and steamed broccoli, cabbage and red pepper

*Turkey burgers with green salad and green beans with garlic and onion

*Grilled fish, pasta salad with zucchini, celery and red pepper

*Salmon souffle with sauce, sauteed cabbage and green salad

*Grilled seafood with green salad and baked potato or steamed broccoli

*Roast turkey or chicken or fish with salad and corn bread

*Grilled salmon or chicken with millet-vegetable salad

*Omelet or quiche (chicken or fish) with green salad

*Broiled salmon with steamed carrots/greens and low-fat yogurt

Vegetable Protein Meals

*Cooked red beans with corn bread and vegetables

*Broccoli, cauliflower and tofu stir fry with green salad

*Tofu and Chinese vegetable salad

*Grain and bean soup with vegetables and crackers

*Tofu/spinach salad with sprouts and whole grain muffin

*Indian spiced beans with green salad and slice millet bread

*Brown rice with tofu and vegetables

*Hearty vegetable/bean stew with side salad and pumpernickel bread

*Tofu or tempeh casserole with brown rice and vegetables

*Vegetable soup with beans; whole grain bread or crackers

*Veggies with tofu garlic cheese

*Baked potato with yogurt and green salad

*Lentil soup with spinach salad and rice crackers

*Brown rice with curried red lentils and salad

*Rice salad with chick pea vegetable spread on rice crackers

*Marinated tofu with vegetable salad

*Baked potato with kefir cheese and salad

*Millet with steamed veggies and light yogurt dressing

*Cole slaw with yogurt dressing, rice and cornbread

*Baked potato casserole with black bean soup and small green salad

*Steamed vegies with tofu dressing and cooked millet

*Vegetarian pizza on toasted chapati

*Light vegetable with whole grain pasta with low fat sauce and green salad

*Whole grain pasta and vegetable casserole

*Vegetable sandwich on whole grain bread with avocado

*Oriental stir fry with bean sprouts, vegies and onion soup

*Vegetable tofu quiche with whole grain crust and mixed greens

*Lentils with carrots, with brown rice or millet burgers and side salad

[1] Mary June Parks, *A New You* (Frankfort, KY: Park Publishers, 1982), p. 24.
[2] H. Leighton Steward, Dr. Morrison C. Bethea, Dr. Samuel S. Andrews, and Dr. Luis A. Balart, *Sugar Busters!* (New York, NY: The Ballantine Publishing Group, 1998), p. 18.
[3] Udo Erasmus, *Fats That Heal/Fats that Kill* (Burnaby, BC: Alive Books, 1993), p. 343.
[4] Brian Scott Peskin, *Beyond the Zone* (Houston, TX: Noble Publishing, 1999), p. 21.
[5] H. Leighton Steward, pp 4-6.

Chapter Summary

- The average American eats 170 pounds of sugar, per person, per year.

- Sugar can make us fat.

- Too many processed carbohydrates can make us fat.

- The wrong fats can make us fat.

- A balanced diet, including protein, good fat, fruits and vegetables, and moderate carbohydrates can help you burn fat.

Motivational Statements:

I love healthy foods. I love fresh fruits and vegetables. I can resist junk foods and candy. Sugar has no power over me.

STEP SIX

Ya Gotta Work Out!

Chapter Thirteen

How To Start an Exercise Program

I grew up when ladies didn't sweat—they perspired. I didn't know a thing about exercise until I was in my mid-20's. When I started, I was really out of shape. I eased into exercise slowly. My first real goal was just to get into a leotard and tights. And even when I was in them, there were parts of me that I wasn't ready to share with the world. I'm so glad the leotard and tights are phasing out to more practical sportswear. They took so long to put on! And it never failed, five minutes after I would put them on, Mother Nature called! (Usually I answer on the first ring.)

Actually I started exercising the minute I began putting on my first pair of leotards. The deep-knee bends and side-to-side motions as I inched and tucked myself into them met all the requirements of a regular workout. Over the past 15 years, though, I have learned how to snow and water ski, play racquetball, run, do aerobics, and lift weights. Not bad for a basically lazy non-exerciser who always tried to get out of gym class. And today I weigh less than I did at age 13.

This section is for you if you: break out into a sweat at even the thought of exercise, consider fighting with the cellophane wrapper on your frozen entree a workout, or pull in your stomach and nothing happens. You might want to go slowly if you are one who buys a tractor mower to cut your 10 foot square lawn.

It's Good for You!

After reading the last chapter, you know that we don't get healthy by exercising alone. And exercise won't help you lose weight if you don't change your diet. Exercise is like the frosting on the cake. But it's no secret that exercise keeps you healthy and slim. Lack of exercise is related to coronary health disease, hypertension, obesity, osteoporosis, and diabetes. Yet not getting enough exercise is a problem for most people. In our complicated, technically advanced society, people have to make the time and effort to exercise.

No matter what level you are on, you can become more fit.

You can win the battle with your body. (If you didn't know there was a battle, just wait until the first day of your exercise program!) How often we complain that we are tired. But we need to take control. If we let it, our body will want to sleep in late, overeat, and never exercise (sounds like the old me!) We have the ability to take control of our bodies. Also, it's easier to be in control of other areas of your life when you first have self-control with your body.

Lots of Benefits

Exercise is one of those things that will help you to get back into the positive Life Cycle of Fitness and victory. It will break you out of that rut. Take a brisk walk outside for 20 minutes and notice how much better you feel. It's good for you for many reasons, and, perhaps, the most important one is your good health.

Exercise is the perfect remedy if you're stressed out, tense, and sluggish. It's one of the best pick-me-ups there is, and is often called a "natural high." I'll warn you, though. Establishing and maintaining an exercise program can be hazardous to your lazy bone. Your life might change. You'll start to watch your diet. You'll care more about your grooming. And you'll keep your home better. Discipline will creep into your life! Oh, no!

Stay Young

Many people think that as we grow older, we automatically gain weight, but I disagree. I weigh less than I did as a teenager. I didn't gain weight throughout my late 40s or early 50s because I was exercising. If you stop exercising, then you lose muscle mass. The more muscle you have, the greater your ability to burn fat. So it's not necessarily age but a slow metabolism that comes from lack of exercise. Regular exercise improves your metabolism and tones your muscles. In fact, the best way to lose weight and stay healthy is through the right diet and regular, aerobic exercise and weight training.

You may discover that it's not just your weight but the lack of exercise that makes you feel fat. I've learned that behind all that flab is a nice muscle just craving to be exposed.

You want muscles. They burn fat. They increase your metabolism. That's why your husband can eat twice as much as you and never gain an ounce. (No fault of his own—he was born with more muscles). Regular exercise helps you get more efficient at burning fat. Some statistics say that you can lose 15 pounds per year by exercising 30 minutes three times a week.

I believe we are more motivated to do things for ourselves when we know the benefits. So, here are 55 benefits to regular exercise to help you convince yourself that it's good for you and worth your time. Exercise helps you(r):

1. Improve your breathing.
2. Improve your circulation.
3. Improve your muscle tone.
4. Decrease your weight.

5. Relieve stress.
6. Spend less time feeling sick.
7. Sleep better.
8. Feel more confident with higher self-esteem and self-worth.
9. Feel more in control of your body.
10. Be more active and productive.
11. Enjoy life with a better attitude.
12. Have more control of your life.
13. Extend your chances of living longer.
14. Have clearer nasal passages.
15. Your skin look more supple.
16. Your ability to burn fat to be more efficient and increase your metabolism.
17. Replace fat with lean tissue; you will lower body fat and lose inches.
18. Combat depression.
19. Lower your blood pressure.
20. Improve your coordination and balance.
21. Normalize/lower your blood sugar.
22. Increase oxygen to the brain which makes you more alert and clear thinking.
23. Decrease your appetite.
24. Increase overall flexibility.
25. Improve your ability to fight disease because your immune system is strengthened.
26. Lower your set point.
27. Reduce the risks of heart disease.
28. Reduce the chance of surviving a heart attack and stroke.
29. Reduce fatigue and increase strength.
30. Improve your posture.
31. Reduce chances of developing varicose veins.
32. Relieve and/or prevent constipation.

33. Decrease your desire for nicotine and other substances.
34. Burn calories more consistently.
35. Strengthen your bones/helps prevent osteoporosis.
36. Remove lactic acid and other poisons from the body.
37. Slow down the aging process.
38. Enjoy a better sex life.
39. Increase your chances of being self-motivated.
40. Improve your relationships.
41. Prevent senility.
42. Achieve lifetime weight control.
43. Increase your HDL cholesterol.
44. Decrease your cancer risk.
45. Improve diabetes management.
46. Lower your resting heart rate.
47. Improve your work performance.
48. Reduce lower back pain.
49. Improve stress management.
50. Reduce anxiety.
51. Increase endurance.
52. Improve your vision.
53. Cleanse the body of toxins.
54. Absolutely improve the overall quality of your life.
55. Have an avenue for a healthy means of escape.

Oxygen Burns Fat

The number-one killer in the United States is cardiovascular disease. Eating a healthy diet is vital to prevent heart disease, but it's also vital to work the heart muscle to get oxygen to the tissues.

Aerobic means "with oxygen." Aerobic exercise means you make a certain amount of demand on your body that is strong enough to get your heartbeat to 70 percent of your maximum heart rate. Additionally, aerobic exercise reduces insulin secretion and increases glucagon secretion, the hormone for fat-burning. And from what we have said about carbohydrates and insulin, it's not a good idea to load up on carbohydrates before aerobic exercise.

The best types of aerobic exercise are: running, walking, jogging, swimming, inline skating, racquetball, cycling, rowing, ice-skating, dancing, tennis, speedwalking, cross-country skiing, aerobic dancing, jazzercize, stair-climbing, skiing, and using a stationary bike or mini trampoline.

Anaerobic exercise, like weight resistance training, helps the body to release one of the best fat burners there is, the human growth hormone. Therefore, combining both aerobic and anerobic exercise can lower fat and increase lean muscle mass.

Exercise raises your metabolism and keeps it raised for several hours after your workout. Most people suggest that to stay at your current level of fitness, exercise three days a week. To improve your fitness, exercise four to six days a week. You need to take a day off every week for your body to rest and recuperate.

There are hundreds of great books and videos on exercise and weight training. In this book, I want to encourage you to get started.

Getting Started

Note: Before you begin any type of exercise program, have a medical examination by a doctor.

1. First, make an appointment with yourself. Get out your calendar right now and mark in three to four days a week that you will exercise, what you will do, and for how long. Look for consistency, not perfection.

2. Go slow. For many people the only exercise they've done recently is running through their mail! Most people

think they have to push and shove their bodies in ways they just can't. But you don't have to do high impact aerobics to make up for lost years.

3. Start with something you like and can do (for a lifetime). Have fun! Experiment. Find a gym. Many people start with walking like I did. When I felt strong enough, I progressed to jogging, then running, and, later, aerobics. Walking briskly is safe and wonderful for just about anyone at any age. Make a commitment and set realistic goals.

4. If you're the kind who needs someone to go with you to stay motivated, then find a partner. Having a friend to workout with will help you stay motivated on the days when you don't feel like working out.

5. Dress right for the weather and get the right pair of shoes. Wear comfortable, cushioned shoes, loose fitting workout clothes, and enjoy yourself. Don't wait until you are slimmer to get proper workout clothes that make you feel good. Look for workout clothes that are made of colors and styles that are flattering at your current weight to keep you motivated.

As for foot gear, when I was a kid, all we had were "sneakers." Today, there are dozens of sophisticated, light weight, form-fitted air-cushioned styles to choose from, which are medically safe (and only cost about one-half of your pay check!)

6. Adjust your attitude. Change your mind about exercise! Don't think about the inconvenience of exercise; think about the results you will be getting. In my weight-loss classes, I have them imagine themselves fit before they even start. I have them see themselves as active people. I take the class for an exercise break and show them my version of power walking. There are two ways to exercise: actively or

passively. The more you put into it, the more you will get out of it. Use those arms and legs and get into it—that's doing it passionately. The thigh is the largest muscle group (you noticed), so you want to work those legs to burn fat. And I recommend that you get some fun music with a beat to keep you going. Make it fun!

7. Enroll in an organized program or have friends join you. Investigate your community resources: the YMCA, parks and recreation department, fitness clubs, local high schools, and colleges. Make it convenient. You won't go to a club that's 40 miles away. Women tend to need more support than men. Women are motivated by friends and family.

8. Determine to stay with it and don't give up. Most people succeed if they stick with it long enough. Focus on your progress and your end results and forget about past mistakes. Do what you can to keep yourself motivated. Plan to do it as a lifestyle.

Find opportunities to be active. Use the stairs instead of the elevator (unless your office is on the 50th floor—you don't want to be late for work and sweaty on top of it all). Take a walk break or lunch instead of those often unproductive coffee breaks.

9. Understand what your goals are and the best way to work out. Be realistic. Find out what your training heartbeat range is (explained later) and try to stay within that range. And be sure to start by stretching for five minutes and warming up for five minutes. (This warns your muscles that you are about to work out!) Stretching prevents injury like shin splints and helps keep your muscles more flexible. Then finish your workout with a five-minute cool down, when you slowly let your heart rate decrease.

Start With Stretching

Stretching is a way to maintain flexibility so you can move fully. Stretching is best done when you finish an aerobic activity like walking or cycling, because your muscles are thoroughly warmed and stretching will be more effective. Stretch all major muscle groups from head to toe before and after each workout.

One thing to remember about stretching is that you want to move slowly and rhythmically, never bounce or jerk. Only do as much as is comfortable. As weeks progress, you will move fuller with less effort.

Walking Is Great Exercise

Walking is easy, safe, cheap, requires no specific equipment, can be done all year round, indoors and outdoors, and, most of all, it's natural. It's the oldest form of exercise known to man (outside of camel riding). It's safe for all ages, less strenuous than other aerobic exercises, and uses almost all of your muscles. Walking is one of the best forms of exercise, especially if you are 30-40 pounds overweight. Just about everyone can walk for 30 minutes. When we don't walk regularly, the circulation slows and the heart has to work harder to make sure enough oxygen reaches the cells in all parts of the body and the waste is removed.

You may be interested in knowing that walking is an excellent way to burn calories. You burn approximately the same calories walking a brisk mile as you do jogging at a leisurely pace. The calories you burn depend more on how far you go or the duration of your exercise session rather than how fast you go. Every mile you walk, you burn approximately 100 calories. A large person burns slightly more, a small person, slightly less.

How To Start Walking

Warm up for 5-10 minutes by walking slowly. As you walk, walk briskly, but moderately. Keep your head up, swing your arms at your sides, taking long strides. This helps your body to be balanced. Start out with 20 minutes for your first mile. As you increase your physical conditioning, increase your pace to 14-15 minutes per mile. The faster you swing your arms, the faster you will walk, as your feet will keep pace with your arm swing. Here are other guidelines: Walk on level ground; hills are too tiring and put demand on the cardiovascular system. Wear clothes that are appropriate for the weather. If warm, wear a cotton sweatsuit; if chilly, wear one or two layers underneath your sweatsuit. Wear a pair of walking or jogging shoes, not tennis shoes. This avoids injury. If you can, go to a place where you can enjoy scenery even if you must drive to get there. For your safety, choose a place where others are exercising. Take a cassette recorder and listen to your favorite tapes.

There have been lots of times during the winter that I wasn't able to get to the health club. One day it was so cold, my car wouldn't even start, and I ended up walking to the grocery store which was a terrific workout. And during the years, I've learned to handle both Thanksgiving and Christmas with "power walks" with the family or friends. Even on my trips out of town to Canada and to visit my Mother in Las Vegas, I was able to stay in shape through walking. You can always get back into the cycle of exercising by just opening the front door and walking!

If you commit to exercising for one year, you can lose 35 pounds of fat. Walking regularly will also keep your body metabolism working. One hour of walking, which equals about three miles, burns from 300-360 calories. One mile can burn 100 calories, and two miles 200 calories (if you are walking a 15 minute or so mile).

Consider Weight Training

I don't have time to train people since I spend so much time with my nutritional practice. But as a personal trainer, I highly recommend weight training to my clients which is becoming more and more popular every year because of it's wonderful benefits. Even the elderly have become fans of resistance training. And it's one of the best ways to burn fat using weights or rubber bands. Aerobic instructors insist that aerobics is the best way to burn fat; and personal trainers insist that weights or resistance training is the best. I think they are both right! Why not incorporate a little of both in your workouts and get the benefit of both? While stretching is done to maintain flexibility, the purpose of resistance training is to increase muscle tone.

If you are just getting into an exercise program, you might give yourself some time to get adjusted to aerobic training, and gradually add weight training. Weight training doesn't mean you have to lift 100 pounds. As a matter of fact, you can get results by using small dumbbells as light as 1-5 pounds every other day. Your own body weight can be used for resistance: as in doing pushups and situps. Take a minimum of 15 minutes three times per week to perform resistance-training exercises.

For fat burning, use the large muscle groups by doing exercises such as squats, bench presses and lateral pulldowns.

When doing any exercises, breathe in during resting phase and exhale during exertion phase. For instance, when performing arm curls, exhale as you lift the weight, inhale as you lower it back down. When doing crunches, exhale as you lift, inhale as you relax and lower shoulders.

For building strength, do between 6-8 repetitions, for toning, do 10-12 repetitions.

Weight training increases bone density, muscle strength, and endurance. The more muscular you are, the higher your metabolic rate and the leaner you can be!

How About Jogging/Running?

You can spot a runner a mile away. They wear special clothes, special shoes, and other special equipment. Like little stop watches or counters, sweatbands, and a walkman. They can't help their love for the sport, because they are addicted, positively. They run with strength and endurance and never seem to mind the neighborhood dogs or shin splints.

Seriously, I absolutely love running! When I warm up and cool down properly, and don't overdo it, I find that it's a safe, effective, and exhilarating workout. It's just a blast! It's best to run on grass or dirt which reduces the stress on the muscular system. I believe running is one of the most natural exercises, too, along with walking.

How Hard, How Long?

If you exercise incorrectly, you will feel wiped out, and you will burn the wrong thing—muscle instead of fat. In fact, if you do feel exhausted after exercising, then you were burning muscle. "No pain, no gain" is not a true statement. People think that the faster and harder the better, but quite the contrary is true. Your goal is to burn fat. Stay in your training zone.

You will need to find your maximum heart rate to know exactly how fast your heart should beat during your 20-30 minute exercise period to get the most out of it. If you don't exercise hard enough, it won't be as effective at burning fat, and if you exercise too hard, you will only wear yourself out.

Here is a simple formula for determining your heart rate range. Find your maximum heart rate. Your maximum heart rate is roughly 220 minus your age (220 - 30 =190). If you are a twenty-year old woman, your maximum heart rate is about 200, if you are forty, it's about 180. The safe range for you is between 40-65% of your maximum heart rate.

To find your ideal heart rate range, find your resting heart rate, or the number of beats of your heart in one minute (when you are resting, take your pulse for 10 seconds and multiply times six). Subtract the number of resting beats per minute from your maximum heart rate which gives you your safe range heart rate. Then multiply this heart rate range by 40-65 and add that answer to your resting heart rate.

For example:

220 Maximum heart rate

-30 Your age

190 Maximum heart rate

-60 Resting heart rate

130 Heart rate range

130 x 40 = 52 + resting heart rate (60) = 112

130 x 65 = 84 + resting heart rate (60) = 144

This ideal heart rate range would be 112 to 144 beats per minute. To see if you are in this range, stop and take your pulse for a minute after you have been running, jogging or walking fast. For example, if you are lower than 112, move faster. If you are higher than 144, slow down.

Exercise When You Don't Want To

When I first started exercising, there were times when I didn't feel like exercising. I would start on a program, and soon my off-days turned into a month. I would always have good reasons for not exercising—like cleaning up around my house, doing the laundry, or washing and waxing the car. After all that, who feels like exercising?

I want to encourage you to get started. Walk for 15 minutes, or around the block like I did when I started. You'll find that as you discipline yourself to walk, you'll walk longer and longer. It will become a positive addiction. Get started and keep it up. You'll reap not only physical but also mental health benefits.

Chapter Summary

- Regular exercise has many benefits.
- Start with stretching.
- Walking is great exercise.
- Consider weight training.
- How About jogging/running?

Motivational Statements:

I love exercise! It's fun and makes me feel great!

STEP SEVEN

Eat at the Right Time

Chapter Fourteen

Are You Really Hungry?

Naturally-thin people used to amaze me. They did unusual things like skip meals when they weren't hungry, or eat only the center of a sub sandwich, leaving the crust. I remember inviting one of my naturally-thin friends to lunch one day. I asked Tammy if she wanted to go right then, at 11:30, or wait until 12:30. Her reply baffled me.

"I'd prefer to wait," she said, "because I'm not hungry yet."

I remember thinking, *So what? What does being hungry have to do with it?*

Tammy's behavior and attitude were opposite from mine. She ate when she was hungry. I could eat any time. She sometimes forgot to eat. I never forgot. In fact, most of the time I remembered only too well, which is why I was the one who was overweight. I thought the only difference between Tammy and me was the fact that she'd been born thin and I had not. I had no idea that her thinking and behavior had as much to do with her weight as her genes.

Tammy thought about food only when it was necessary to eat. Until I changed my thinking and behavior, I thought about food all the time. *To every thing there is a season, and a time* (Ecc. 3:1). As far as eating went, anytime was the right time for me! Since then, I've learned how to trust my body's signals.

Food is Everywhere

This change was not easy. There were so many reasons why I wanted to think about food and eat. For example, pick up a recent copy of any woman's magazines and you'll find dozens of recipes, diets and ideas about how to eat. The reason most diets don't work is because they're not designed around how your body burns fat.

Still today, I'm reminded of my old behavior when I meet people who begin thinking about lunch just as soon as they finish breakfast. While some thought about food is necessary, too much thinking about food becomes an obsession.

Hunger Is Natural

Eating at the right time means eating when it's natural for your body. You're hungry. You want to eat.

Hunger is a signal that tells your body you need more food. If you eat when you're not hungry, your body knows you don't need more food, so it does the only logical thing it can do—it stores the excess as fat!

Never get upset with your body for what it's doing. It's only doing what it was designed to do. Your body is your friend, because you are fearfully and wonderfully made (Ps. 139:14).

Often you can tell whether or not you are actually hungry by *what* you are craving. If you are craving Twinkies and M&Ms, it's a good indication that it's not a true physical hunger. True physical hunger causes cravings for healthy food, like an apple.

Where Is It Written?

As a nutritionist, I believe in good nutrition and eating a balanced diet. But how much is really enough? Most guidelines are meant for averages, like the average man or average woman. Then we have to consider their size, weight and activity, and individual metabolism. But who said we need to eat 3 meals and 2 snacks? In the early 70s, while doing research, I discovered that there were other guidelines for eating. There was a Basic 12 Food Group, then the Basic

Seven, and later some of you might remember the Basic Four food groups. Now we have the Food Pyramid. Who wrote these? What were they based on? None of them were based on any clinical studies, especially our current guidelines.

In her book, *The Diet Alternative*, Diane Hampton says the Bible pattern was only two meals a day. I've found that works for many people. Especially if their first meal is breakfast, they eat a good lunch, and maybe some fruit for dinner; not another large meal. Why make someone eat three times when they are only hungry for two meals? (As long as one of the meals isn't a coffee and a donut!) Sometimes I think people can get confused and eat too much if we tell them they need to eat three meals. I like to see how my clients feel on a three meal a day plan. If they've only eaten two meals all their life, why should I change it now? Everyone is different. Perhaps eating only twice might help them to know their real hunger signals and help them lose weight.

(Of course, if you have a blood-sugar problem, it might be harder for you to only eat twice.)

Benefits of Eating at the Right Time

Why be concerned about eating only when you're really hungry? Obviously, to lose weight. Overeating, even protein foods, causes a higher insulin level which sets up a cycle of food cravings and storing fat. Here are other benefits.

You will have/be:

1. Stable blood-sugar level
2. Increased energy levels for new activities
3. Fewer mood swings
4. Less fat stored
5. Healthier skin, flatter stomach
6. No feeling of being deprived

7. More in touch with body

8. More enjoyment of foods

9. Less dependent on external controls

10. Freedom from the dieting cycle

11. No more food-obsessions

12. Stronger spiritually

We can trust our body's natural hunger/full signals when we are eating right. I don't mean we're hungry because we ate pancakes or Belgium waffles for breakfast so now we crave more foods, or hunger because we're bored and looking for something to do—like eat. But real hunger. But we often are making mistakes that hinder us from knowing our body's natural hunger signals. Let's look at some.

1. We Eat Too Late at Night

Many clients say their greatest challenge is eating too late at night. They find that after dinner it's too easy to raid the refrigerator and grab a snack.

If we eat a certain number of calories, say 1200, but we eat them all just before bed, we will gain more weight than the person who eats the same amount of calories, but eats them throughout the day. And in chapter 12, I said that if you eat too many starches and not enough protein, you may find yourself craving starches all night. Try eating some protein with vegetables and a small starch at dinner, or skip the evening carbohydrate serving.

2. We Skip Breakfast

You've heard that it's ideal to eat a big breakfast, small lunch, and light dinner. Eating too late in the evening dulls the appetite for breakfast. So eat light at night and heavier in the daytime. Once you re-train your body to these new signals, you will become hungry for breakfast every morning. In fact, a good rule of thumb is, if your largest meal is breakfast, you will lose weight, if your largest meal is lunch you will maintain your weight, and if your largest meal is dinner, you will gain weight.

3. We Skip Meals

The idea of meal-skipping for weight loss is counter-productive. What usually happens is that we make up the missing food later in the day. You can't help it. Your body expects a certain number of calories and it will get them one way or another!

Eating food increases your metabolism. That means when you are not eating, your metabolism slows down so you stop burning fat and stop losing weight.

Remember though, that eating too many carbohydrates or sugars will raise your circulating insulin which will make you feel hungry, too. How can you really be hungry when you just ate a large meal? You're not—you only feel like you are because of the insulin.

It may take awhile to get in touch with true hunger signals. The best way to follow your signals is to design your life so that you eat three or four small meals a day, training yourself to sense and know your body's signals. When hunger strikes, you can plan to eat something healthy instead of desperately searching for a vending machine.

Why Diets Don't Work

Bob Schwartz wrote an interesting book called *Diets Don't Work* with a revision, *Diets Still Don't Work* many years ago. Bob found that many of people's problems regarding food were not just about food. And he presented the idea of gauging your hunger. This might help you. You might not have thought about this, but we can trust our body's hunger/full signals to tell us if we need food. If we're hungry, then we'll use the food that we eat. If we're continually eating but we're not really hungry, then we'll probably store the excess as fat.

Rate your hunger on a scale of one to ten, with ten being stuffed and filled to the brim, so much that you can't eat anymore. Number one means you are empty and legitimately hungry. We'll look more at the full side of this gauge in chapter 16. For now, let's focus on knowing when you are hungry.

Hunger Gauge

1. empty, legitimately hungry (lose weight)
2. ready for fuel
3. tolerable, but hungry
4. slightly, somewhat hungry
5. satisfied
6. past feeling satisfied
7. slightly uncomfortable gain weight
8. more than full
9. very, very full
10. stuffed, filled to the brim, beyond my limit

People lose weight here   People gain weight here

1____2____3____4____5____6____7____8____9___10___

empty ready tolerable slightly hungry satisfied past uncomfortable full very full stuffed

Each of us can rate our hunger and the size of our stomach according to this scale. Stop now for just a moment and squeeze your hand into a fist. Look at your fist. This is the normal size of your stomach. At point number one, when you are truly hungry, your stomach is the size of your fist. At point number ten, you are stuffed beyond your limit. Now your stomach has increased two or three times its original size to accommodate the overload of food. The stomach is trying its best to accommodate what you are giving it!

But don't wait till you are so famished that your body is weak and wobbling from lack of glucose in the blood. But it is good to wait till you are comfortably hungry, which ranges from points one-to-three. The less hungry you are, the less you want to eat. The mistake most overweight people make, is to eat at point four when they are only slightly hungry, just as they would at point one when they are very hungry. The result is weight gain!

A good rule of thumb is to wait until you are genuinely hungry, (at points 1 and 2) and eat until you are satisfied (point 5). Most eating after point 5 will—you guessed it—end up on your hips, thighs and tummy. To further help, you might want to use the Hunger Chart at the end of this chapter. Mark H for hungry, S for satisfied, or F for full to become aware of your hunger patterns. Try it for a week.

Too Busy to Eat Right?

People are in such a rush going to and from work, appointments, and social engagements, there's often no time to eat properly. So plan ahead. Get some substitutes. Great snacks are protein snacks like boiled eggs, natural cheese or raw almonds or sunflower seeds.

If healthy substitutes are not readily available, you will end up running into the local convenience store and grabbing a cup of coffee and a chocolate donut. This in turn puts you back into the downward spiral of the quick fix and later weight gain.

Why Are You Eating?

Another aspect of eating at the right time is eating for the right reasons. Some people who don't have much to do, may spend a lot of time buying, preparing and eating food. Food is more than just a necessity, it has become a full-time job!

Another reason why people eat when they don't need to is the inability to say "No thank you," when they're not hungry. Perhaps you can practice "speaking the truth in love" the next time your Aunt Mabel pushes her Boston cream pie on you when you are already full. Perhaps you can accept one piece and then take it home with you and pop it into the freezer.

What happens when you come home from work? Too hungry to wait to eat? Do you gobble down all your snacks before dinner? I used to do that. Then, I'd get hungry again and want to eat dinner! No wonder I was overweight!

One trick that helps me deal with the transition time between coming-home and supper, is to take a moment and put on some music, rather than running right to the refrigerator. I found that I can deal with this time easier with good music than with food. If I'm too hungry to fix dinner, I eat a piece of fruit instead of bingeing on high-fat foods.

You understand about eating when you are hungry. You know what foods to eat, but you sometimes just eat for no reason. Let's look next at why we eat.

Chapter Summary

- You can trust your body's signals for hunger.
- Getting in touch with your own hunger and full signals will help in weight control.
- Eating several small meals aids in losing weight.
- Using the Hunger Gauge will assist you in knowing when you are genuinely hungry.

Motivational Statements:

I eat when I'm hungry. I love natural foods. It's easy to know my natural body signals.

Hunger Chart

H=Hungry   S=Satisfied   F=Full

Date	Breakfast	Snack	Lunch	Snack	Dinner	Snack

Chapter Fifteen

Why Do You Eat?

When I was trying to lose weight, I would plan my meals. I'd eat a good breakfast, a good lunch and light dinner. My goal was not to eat after 7:00 at night. I remember one night having dinner with friends. I thought, *Well, I'm not that hungry, but I'll have a bite to eat.* I found myself eating the whole dinner, rolls, and dessert! Then later that night, a friend, Andy and I went to a movie. Andy got popcorn, so I ate popcorn. And I wasn't even hungry! Where did all of my resolve not to eat go?

Our eating can be so automatic. We can forget that our habits are made of small behaviors that are tied to eating. We eat because something triggers the response. It may be the good taste of food. Do you know anyone who can walk into a movie theater and not want a big box of hot-buttered popcorn? The smell of popcorn and the association of good times can trigger popcorn cravings! (Are they using real butter, or is it just a great butter-flavored aroma therapy?)

Or it may be because of what your parents told you, such as, "Clean your plate," "Eat all your veggies," and "There are starving children in Africa."

What Makes Us Eat?

Lots of things. You may want to eat when you're with certain people, like going out to dinner. Or when you are at a certain location, like Star Bucks. Or during a certain activity, like shopping. We work up such an appetite! Even certain emotions can send people to the refrigerator. And they don't have to be negative emotions. Some people eat when they're sad, and when they're happy.

Or, you might eat when you are under stress. You use food to relax because certain types of foods, carbohydrates, for example, can cause you to feel more relaxed.

Some people associate behavior patterns with food. Perhaps your mother gave you a cookie when you were good. Now you're conditioned to want something sweet when you feel you deserve it. Food has become your *reward*.

One of my clients named Dr. Nanette Lane is the Principal of Coweta Central Elementary School. Her comment to me was, "How many of us got candy for rewards in school? How many of us stop to think as adults, that getting candy for rewards could have set us up for some eating patterns later in life?" Dr. Lane is looking at how they can find alternatives to using food for rewards.

All of these are food triggers which means they set off a *trigger* which makes you want to eat. There are a wide variety of circumstances which set off food triggers in our minds. As with knowing our thoughts, we have to know our patterns before we can break them. That sounds easy enough. It's just that some of these patterns are unconscious and automatic— like tying your shoes and brushing your teeth. You just do them without thinking.

I used to write in a Food Diary and I tell my clients to do it too. Did you know it's hard to remember the food you ate when you eat it in the dark? Like the popcorn at the movie theater? Amazing how often that is forgotten!

So we have to know what in the world we are really doing before we can change our habits. Then we can start somewhere, and break one pattern at a time.

How Did Mom and Dad Eat?

What kind of patterns did you learn from your family? Sometimes it helps to remember how you were raised. Did your family snack a lot? Did they eat out a lot? Look at this list and think about what you did as a family and what you are doing now. Any similarities?

Did your mother serve large portions?

Did your family eat high-fat foods?

Did your family eat while doing things like reading and watching television?

Did they use sweets to celebrate holidays?

Did they have snacks like popcorn at night or candy bars often?

Did they often eat at restaurants?

Did they eat on the run?

How often did they eat at home?

Did they eat to handle stress or deal with emotions?

This list might help you to see how much your family's influence has affected your eating patterns. Don't criticize yourself or your family after doing this exercise. Just be aware of your patterns. You're a step closer to knowing what to change.

Types of Triggers

When I taught my weight-loss class, I asked people to tell me when, why and where they were when they wanted to eat. The list below is what we came up with. You may want to add a few of your own. The categories were emotional triggers (like when they were upset or stressed), activity triggers (watching TV); location triggers (a certain place or location makes you want to eat); social triggers (certain people may trigger you to eat); food triggers (Drinking a soda makes you want French fries); or physical triggers (hunger or stress).

1. Emotional Triggers

Not getting what you want
Procrastinating
Holding back thoughts and feelings
Boredom
Seeking pleasure
Attempting to avoid feelings
Feeling emotionally empty

2. Activity Triggers

Watching television
Watching a movie
While working
Working on the computer
Working on craft projects
Writing letters
Reading the newspaper
Reading the Bible
Bowling
Playing cards
Traveling in the car

3. Location Triggers

At a movie
In the car
In the den
In the living room
Near the refrigerator
At desk at work
In the bedroom
On the couch
At a particular coffee shop or restaurant

At a sales meeting or in the office break room
While grocery shopping
While putting groceries away

4. Social Triggers

Going out with friends
Going to a movie
Going to brunch
Going shopping
Going out for dessert
Going to another person's house for dinner
Going to a banquet
Thanksgiving, Christmas and other holidays
Anniversaries, birthdays

5. Food Triggers

Salt
Sugar
Caffeine, sodas, coffee
Popcorn
Ice cream
Hot dogs
Sausage

6. Physical Triggers

Hunger
Stress

What Will The Future Hold?

Wouldn't it be nice if we could have more technology to help us know how much to eat? Like, a buzzer goes off on our belt if we are over our caloric limit for the day! Or, when you go to a restaurant, a machine records your cholesterol results before you can order dessert!

As long as the food industry makes tantelizing commercials, we're going to have to be aware of these triggers. There was a time when just seeing the banana split with the chocolate fudge dripping over it made me jump in the car and drive down to the neighborhood Braum's. Now I don't even think about ice cream. I've changed my reaction to food triggers.

Once you start noticing triggers for eating, you'll notice they're everywhere! We get dozens of cues every day. And look at our holidays. Each one has food attached to it. New Year's Day brunch, Valentine's Day candy, Easter chocolates, Halloween candy, Thanksgiving dinner, and Christmas parties and dinner. Then throw in a few anniversary and birthday parties. There will always be reasons to celebrate, and Americans love to celebrate with food!

Every day we get scores of invitations to eat, from billboards, television, radio, magazines and newspapers. So if you're waiting for outside circumstances to change, nothing will ever happen. You must take control!

You Can Say, "No"

Did you know you don't have to eat when you're under stress? I know people who never eat when they're stressed. I also know people who never eat popcorn at the movies. They can pass by a bakery and not run inside and make a purchase. They are conditioned that way. You can be too! Let's look at a tool to help you that I call a Trigger Chart (See page 203).

Know What You Are Doing

The first step in using the Trigger Chart is becoming aware of when you are eating. Write down three or four of your eating situations and then write down one of the six triggers. Go down the list one by one, beginning with breakfast. Were you really hungry? Then it was a physical trigger, so write a "P" in the box. How about a mid-morning snack? What triggered you to eat it? It may have been an emotional trigger, so write in "E." And what about the foods that trigger overeating such as chips, salted nuts, popcorn? All of these "night" snacks may be food triggers ("F"), as well as activity ("A") triggers.

Once you have recorded these patterns you have taken the first step toward identifying food triggers. After evaluating, then you can break the patterns as we have already explained in previous chapters. Your main goal is to learn to eat when you are really hungry. Then you can eat what you enjoy in a portion you know will nourish you. Life isn't about food. Don't let food be the only way to celebrate your life or handle your emotions.

Pickles Anyone?

The second step is to write down how you will deal with these various situations. Think of another way to handle the situation. What else could you do besides eat? Or maybe you could change the food. When I lived in Portland, Oregon, we used to go to a movie theatre that offered pickles along with the usual popcorn. Surprisingly, I got so I preferred my pickle to a bowl of popcorn.

So find a substitute for the food or behavior. You'll be stopping one pattern by replacing it with another—making new brain imprints.

Modify Your Behavior

Behavior modification is a fancy term which means consciously changing your association between the food and activity. Once that happens, you'll find that the "automatic" need to eat no longer controls your life. Here are some ideas.

1. No, I Don't Want Bread or Chips and Salsa!

I used to eat and then eat again. First, I'd eat bread or chips and salsa and then I'd eat dinner. Since it's hard to resist food sitting right in front of you, tell the waiter to hold the snacks! (Give yourself a fighting chance for dessert!)

2. Purposely Leave Food

I know that people are starving everywhere. Mom told us, remember? I was taught to clean up my plate. Were you? But I learned to leave food on my plate, too. Or, just split a sandwich, like my friend Anne and I do often. We save money that way, too. Or, just box it up and take it home. It's okay to eat less. Give money to your favorite charity of loaves and fishes.

3. Pack It Up! Quick!

I used to eat dinner and go to the kitchen to put my plate away. When I saw the rest of the food sitting there in the pan, I took another helping! Sometimes I ate it all. Ouch! Wish I had just put it away. So I've learned to cook what I need and put the rest away as quickly as possible!

4. Replace Junk Foods

If it's out of sight, it will be out of mind. I've actually forgotten that I had a great piece of carrot cake (my favorite if I ever eat desserts) in the back of the refrigerator until it was too late. The mold had four colors! Have nuts and apples around. They're safer.

5. Eat At a Specific Place

At home or work have a specific place to do all your eating. At home, eat at the dinner table. At work, eat at the break room, not your desk.

6. Shop With a List

Just a few things about shopping: Shop with a list when you go, and don't send your spouse if they are not health conscious! Not unless you want Fruit Loops, Chips Ahoy and popcorn! I've noticed that most men are not natural nutritionists. It's not natural for them to stop and consider, "How much sugar is in this product? Let's see..." No, like they shop for clothes, they are used to just running and grabbing. This behavior must have come from generations ago when man ran after wild game, shot or killed it and dragged it home. Life was so simple then!

It's not always easy to use a chart like this. Sometimes it's easier to wear loose-fitting clothing and control top panty hose! But after using this chart a couple of weeks, you'll finally know why in the world you are eating. Great, that's your first step to change. Never mind how often, or where. Take one habit and make it a goal. Put it on your Life Design Planning Chart. And change one of them at a time.

Chapter Summary

- There are a wide variety of circumstances which set off food triggers in our minds.

- Your family's eating history will help to identify your food triggers.

- Use a chart to identify triggers and to be set free from their control.

- Modify your behavior.
    1. No, I don't want bread or chips and salsa!
    2. Purposely leave food.
    3. Pack it up! Quick!
    4. Replace junk foods.
    5. Eat at a specific place.
    6. Shop with a list.

Motivational Statement:

I know when I eat and I only eat when my body needs food.

Trigger Chart

E=Emotional   A=Activity   L=Location
S=Social   F=Food   P=Physical

Date	Breakfast	Snack	Lunch	Snack	Dinner	Snack

STEP EIGHT

Eat the Right Portion

Chapter Sixteen

You Don't Have To Eat It All!

It wasn't always easy for me to know when to stop eating. Perhaps it's the microwaves. All I have to do is open the door of my microwave oven, set a healthy meal on the turntable and four minutes later it's time to eat! In another two minutes it's all eaten. (It's not like I have to go out and pluck the chickens!) Unfortunately, according to research, it takes fourteen more minutes for my brain to get the message that I've already eaten. And as you are well aware, a person can eat a lot more food in fourteen minutes.

How much do you really need to eat? Can't zip up last year's jeans? You're eating more than you did last year. How much more?

Our economy may be downsizing, but we're not! The U.S. Department of Agriculture says that 58 million Americans are overweight. And only 26 percent of Americans meet the daily dietary recommendations for dairy, and fewer than 20 percent eat the recommended two to three servings of fruit. I've even had clients ask, "What's a fruit again?"

In the past twenty years, our daily calories have gone from about 1850 to 2000. But that 150 calories a year adds up to about 15-20 pounds a year.

What's up? We're eating more and we don't even realize it.

Think about it. When I was a teenager, McDonald's had 6 to 8 ounces of soft drinks. Today, cans hold from 12 ounces to a half liter.

We're all eating too much, even children. Ten percent of children are overweight, and 70 percent of those children will become obese as adults.

Serving sizes on the Food Pyramid don't match nutritional labels on products. Juice used to be served in a 4-5 ounce glass; today we feel jipped if we don't get a 8-10 ounce glass. And dinner plates, which used to be around 8 inches are now 10-12 inches. Restaurants boast about how much food you get—as much as thirty percent more in the last ten years. No wonder we are confused. No wonder we are overweight. We hear about what a portion is and then we go to a restaurant and eat one and a half to three times that amount! We just don't know what a portion is anymore.

We're eating more and enjoying it less! We are out of touch with our own body signals, and we have lost the taste for natural foods that God has provided. There are several reasons why we are so out of touch. Let's look at a few.

1. We Eat Junk Food

A malnourished body cries out for good food, but instead of whole foods, you feed it non-foods such as Twinkies, potato chips, candy bars, and soda pop. Hmmm, where's the protein, B vitamins, minerals and good fat there? Afterward, the body is still hungry because no *nourishment* has been registered. Your body says, "Wait a minute! We haven't eaten anything significant yet. Eat more." Many people try to live on junk food, and as a result their bodies are undernourished. The body will continue to send out hunger signals and the person will never understand why they can't get "full."

2. We Have Poor Digestion

Due to poor digestion from eating so many processed foods, our bodies may not be absorbing proper nutrients. When no nutrients are being absorbed, our body sets off an alarm that it has not been fed, causing us to want to eat more. Get some digestive enzymes and read my other book.

207

3. We Are Trained to Overeat

Everywhere we go, we are encouraged and even *trained* to eat too much. From Sunday brunch at Grandma's to the lavish all-you-can-eat buffets, fats and calories scream at us to tempt and cajole us to partake. After all, we paid for it all! We want to get our money's worth. Even if it doesn't show up on our well-toned thighs (and it often does), overeating will take a dangerous toll on the heart! Of course, we can afford to overeat, while those in third-world countries cannot. (Could this be why our life span is shorter than theirs?) When my sister, Jackie, and her husband lived in South Africa I made several visits to their home. In Africa, I noticed that people ate and were satisfied with smaller meals. There was little obesity because they couldn't afford it.

4. We Wait Too Long Between Breakfast and Lunch

Our national problem with overeating could be due to our tradition of eating breakfast comprised of sugar and/or carbohydrates. We try to wait three to five hours for lunch. By that time, we're famished and tired. When we do eat, then we tend to overeat to make up for it. Meanwhile, we've lost our ability to know when we are really full.

Other cultures, on the other hand, eat more often. I once lived in West Germany for nearly three years, and traveled around Europe during that time. Europeans eat five or six small meals during the day. Our grandparents, Oma and Opa were in better shape than I was; I gained 30 pounds!

Diabetics have known for years that more frequent meals stabilize the release of insulin needed to keep the blood-sugar level stable. Eating smaller meals discourages overeating since eating like this doesn't overfill the stomach. Remember, in the last chapter we established that our stomach's natural size is no bigger than our fist.

5. We Eat For Emotional Reasons

Many people eat to deal with their emotions. They may feel bored, or upset, or frightened. By eating something, they know they will feel better. Use the tools in this book, and consider Christian counseling if you fall in this category and nothing you have tried helps.

6. We Think There's Not Enough Food to Go Around

There's yet another emotional bond to eating and that is the fear of never having enough. Or that we may never get to eat again. Absurd, isn't it? But these unconscious thought patterns may stem from childhood experiences when there was a genuine lack of food, and the emotions can be deeply imbedded in our subconscious minds.

For those overeaters who experience such a fear, there are ways to conquer this fear. As a former compulsive overeater, I am very familiar with the thought pattern: *I've just got to have this food now.*

You can get rid of a lot of these patterns by just following a healthy balanced diet and learn all you can about cravings and nutrition.

Another way to quiet this fear is to practice leaving food on your plate. Begin with leaving just a few bites. Then try leaving a little bit more. By doing this, you are telling your subconscious mind that you *know* there is more coming. This again, strikes at the core of the fear that there is not enough.

But past that, think about this country we live in and the abundance that surrounds us. If you run out of food, you can go down to the grocery store, day or night and buy more. If that's not convenient enough, you can find fast-food restaurants on almost every corner.

I used to love desserts, and I especially loved Tiramisu, an Italian version of cheesecake. Every time I ate at an Italian restaurant, I had to have this rich dessert even though I was already stuffed and knew I didn't need another bite. The way I conquered this problem is by doing what I've explained here. I simply told myself I could have it another time. Literally, I would talk myself out of it. I found I no longer wanted Tiramisu at all. Now I rarely, if ever, order any dessert, let alone Tiramisu.

Had Enough Yet?

Earlier in chapter 14 we had you think about when you're hungry. Now I want you to think about when you're full. Full means you don't need to eat any more. I used to think that full meant stuffed.

As I trained myself to stop eating the moment I felt comfortably full, and did it on a regular basis, I began to lose weight.

If you have trouble with overeating, don't eat so many carbohydrates and sugar and eat smaller meals. Large heavy meals cause a greater demand on your digestion system and cause quick weight gain.

At first, I had difficulty adjusting to eating less. I remember thinking, *Is this all I get?* I felt uneasy eating smaller meals— I wanted more. I had been overeating for so long, I needed time to get used to smaller portions.

You too may experience a period of adjustment as you move out of your comfort zone. Any time you want to change a habit, you can expect a time of uneasiness until you establish the new habit. With time, your stomach will return to its normal size and you will then become accustomed to smaller amounts of food.

More Tips

1. Buy proportioned plates like picnic plates and eat only the portion allowed.

2. Buy nutritious frozen dinners to become accustomed to what a normal portion is for most people. The first few times I tried this, it was difficult. I added bread or a salad to convince myself I had enough. Now, the dinner alone is enough.

3. Planning is essential. Knowing you get to eat again in a couple of hours gives you permission to eat a small amount now. This knowledge frees you from the fears often associated with not getting to eat. You can eat smaller meals with joy and peace.

4. Eating the right types of foods will help you not overeat. Highly sweetened or salted foods stir up cravings and binges. Eating healthy food is always better. The more you eat nutritious food, the less likely you will crave junk food.

5. Fast some meals or days. Just don't eat if you're not hungry. If you eat too much one day, then eat light the next day. Read books on fasting. Fast a day every week with herbal teas, and popular green drinks, like Barley Green. Green foods are cleansing and building. You can find out more about these at your health food store. (Only water fast with a doctor's supervision.) The healthier you are, the easier fasting becomes. Make it a great health and weight-loss tool.

From Fast Foods to Whole Foods

Eating whole foods high in nutrition will result in eating less food but higher quality food. Whole foods will leave you feeling satisfied. I like to eat natural foods. I experience higher energy levels from a more nutritious diet. Having energy is a wonderful feeling!

It's not the one time that you overeat that puts on weight, it's the continual overeating. We fall into a trap when we overeat one time and it sets off bingeing. Instead of looking at it as a one-time slip-up, we write off the whole morning, afternoon, evening, week, month or year! This attitude puts us back in the negative Diet Cycle.

One slip-up doesn't mean you've lost the whole battle. There's a way to handle occasional lapses. If you eat heavy on one day, take control as quickly as possible. Recognize that you are out of control. Use the principles in this book. Wait until you are hungry again by recognizing the body signals. Soon you'll be right back on track once again.

As you begin to follow your body's signals—eating when you are physically hungry, stopping when you have had a sufficient amount, and eating healthy foods—you will feel satisfied. Feeding your body only when it is hungry means your body won't go into a starvation mode and store fat. Thus, you will break the dieting cycle and you will gradually lose your interest in overeating and in junk food. You'll get and stay in the Life Cycle of Fitness.

Chapter Summary

- We're eating more and enjoying it less!
- Why are we so out of touch with our natural body signals?
  1. We eat junk food.
  2. We have poor digestion.
  3. We are trained to overeat.
  4. We wait too long to eat.
  5. We eat for emotional reasons.
  6. We think there's not enough food.

Motivational Statements:

I eat just what's right for me. It's easy to stop when I'm full.

Chapter Seventeen

What Are You Really Eating?

What did you eat for dinner last night? The night before? Last Tuesday? Have you forgotten already? Unless we write down small details like these, they are easily forgotten—except for a special celebration pizza or a mud-pie ice-cream dessert! Who can forget those?

The foods you choose determine your health and your weight. What you eat matters; it all adds up. For example, it's logical to think, *What can one cookie, one piece of pie, or one bowl of ice cream matter?*

The problem is that every time you eat sugar, your insulin rises, and stays high for awhile—perhaps a day or two. That one dessert, or cookie that you eat every day could be the one thing that keeps you from losing weight.

You Can't Eat It All

Have you ever seen a sign or ad that told you that you could eat everything you wanted and still lose weight? Well, you can't. Not unless you want to go against how your body is made, and mess up your digestion, or fat metabolism. But you can change how you eat. Change starts with knowing what, how much, and when you eat.

What Are You Eating?

In order to change your eating habits, you have to start associating the foods you are choosing right now with your current weight. What you eat now—today—is causing your current level of weight and quality of health. You will take control of your eating habits only when you become aware of the types and amounts of food you eat.

That's why monitoring your behavior with the Food Diary is so effective! (See page 219). Keeping a daily record of everything you eat and drink can be the first step to change. Don't skip this important step! After counseling thousands of people, the ones who worked with a diary found weight loss easier and were more successful at losing and keeping it off.

In fact, when people look at me and say that they won't use one, or don't want to fill out the food diary, that usually means that they just aren't serious about weight loss. They don't want to know what in the world they're doing! You can't change what you don't know needs changing.

Why is This Valuable?

This may be the first time in your life that you will become acutely aware of your daily eating patterns. Instead of wondering how many times you've had dessert this week, or how many times you chose to eat a salad, you will have the record right there in front of you.

Without a Food Diary, it's so easy to eat unconsciously. You grab the bag of potato chips out of the cupboard and sit down to watch television. You were only going to eat a few chips, but before you know it, the entire package is empty. An hour later, you get up from the couch, look at the bag and wonder, *When did I eat the whole thing?*

What Happens?

Two things will happen when you keep a Food Diary. First, you will see the amount proteins, fats, carbohydrates, fruits and vegetables you consume. Secondly, you will become aware of your eating patterns. The most effective way to increase your awareness is to keep a record of when you eat, where you were, what you were doing, if you were hungry, and if you overate. Photocopy this chart and use it daily for at least a week.

Once you begin to see the patterns of when you "blew it," you can take action to prevent it from happening as often. And likewise, as you begin to see where you are successful in saying no to temptation, and making healthy eating choices, you are encouraged in your journey toward weight loss and better health.

I Could Have Had an Olive!

Remember the television commercial that said, "Wow! I could have had a V8!" You could choose four carrot or cucumber sticks rather than four chocolate chip cookies! I've learned to have something else, like an olive or pickle.

How can you change something if you don't know what needs changing? Keeping a Food Diary shows you how you got out of shape and will help motivate you to get back into shape. The Food Diary forces us to get blatantly honest with ourselves. We must admit how often and how much we eat.

Your diary will show how often you eat during the course of a day: three, four, five or even six times. Eating more frequently isn't a bad thing if you are eating small, healthy meals. But what are you eating, and what size portions? Do you eat at home or do you frequent the restaurants? Do you go out and eat for entertainment several times a week? Do you eat with someone?

By using your diary you'll see if you eat more on the weekends than during the week, or if you habitually snack on junk food when you come home from work. You will see how often you eat from emotional hunger rather than physical hunger, and how often you stop when you are full.

Be Honest

Don't be afraid to record when you overate, or when you ate but were not really hungry. You are looking for patterns, not perfection. The Food Diary will help track your triumphs as well as your failures. What about the time you were able to resist a donut at the office? When everyone else is enjoying the jelly-filled and chocolate-covered donuts in the break room, it can be one of the hardest times to resist. Give yourself credit for that one!

So get out your pen and start writing. Write down everything you eat and drink over the course of the next week. As you are writing, make note of the types of foods that you eat, whether raw or cooked.

At the end of the week, take time to study the patterns. It's time to get brutally honest with yourself. Do you see obvious patterns that can be changed now? Are you eating right after supper? Is the sugar intake higher than what you thought? Perhaps you've been able to cut out a few cups of coffee during the week. Jot down these patterns.

Keep this diary and use it whenever you want to get back in control of your eating.

Benefits of the Food Diary
You Know What You Eat

Keeping a Food Diary forces you to take a hard, honest look at the food choices you make every day. Suddenly, you will become sharply aware of what you are eating. In fact, failure to use a Food Diary or similar tool, may mean you will not succeed in changing your behavior. Like a bowler who never became aware of her first step, it can greatly affect your final outcome.

Are you getting enough good nutrition every day? The Food Diary will show where you're lacking. Fill in the circles at the bottom of the chart. Perhaps your diet lacks sufficient fruits (1 to 2 per day) and veggies (at least one salad and one serving of steamed vegetables per day), or not enough intake of water. Likewise, the diary will indicate if too much coffee or sugar is depleting the nutrients in your body.

You Know How Much You Eat

Most people have no idea of the amount of food they eat. Portion control is vital in weight loss. A person may be eating the right foods, but eating too much. Writing it down will help to chart these patterns as well.

You Know When You Eat

Do you eat consistently throughout the day, or do you find that you eat everything at night—a sure way to gain weight!

You Know Why You Eat

What sends you running to the fridge for chocolate chip ice cream? Does boredom cause you to want to grab the potato chips? Is stress driving you to binge? In this case, you might want to also use the Trigger Chart.

If you want, you can ease slowly into using the Food Diary. For the first week, record what you eat to discover your eating patterns. On the second week, use the chart to figure out fat grams, calories and portion sizes.

A word of caution. Never let one little downfall cause you to throw away the Food Diary. No one is perfect. Perhaps you overate one day, or ate the wrong foods. Using the diary will help you to see the mistake, and it will guide you back on track. The exciting moment will come when you look back over your chart and see there are fewer and fewer of these downfalls.

Chapter Summary

- Monitoring behavior through use of the Food Diary will give an honest picture of eating patterns.
- Benefits of the Food Diary
  1. You know what you eat.
  2. You know how much you eat.
  3. You know when you eat.
  4. You know why you eat.
- Don't let one little downfall cause you to stop using the Food Diary

Motivational Statements:

It's easy to use a Food Diary. It helps me know what I'm eating.

Life Design Food Diary

Name _____

Weight/Size Goal _____

	MONDAY	TUESDAY	WEDNESDAY	THURSDAY	FRIDAY	SATURDAY	SUNDAY
Breakfast							
Snack							
Lunch							
Snack							
Dinner							
Snack							

Chapter Eighteen

Never Give Up!

In this book, we have looked at two parts to change: the mental side and the physical side. We've seen the eight steps to change, starting with a firm foundation for change, which included understanding change, changing your thoughts, finding your motivation, and planning your life.

Then we looked at the fat-burning foods, exercise, eating at the right time, and eating the right amounts of food. All of these steps are valuable for permanent weight loss.

You are learning about making lifestyle changes in your life that, if you continue to do them, will help you lose weight and keep it off this time. The people who succeed at anything in life are those who continue to keep going in the right direction. They are the ones who keep on keeping on, and never give up! To keep moving forward you have to keep reminding yourself of your picture. Keep imagining yourself looking, acting, and feeling differently. Help yourself to get and stay motivated. You can do that with your words.

Below is a review of many motivational phrases that I have used to keep myself motivated. You saw these first in chapter 8. Additionally, I have reviewed all of the motivational statements from each of the chapters of the book in the Appendix.

Find statements that encourage you, or move you to action and keep them before you. That way you will never give up, and the fat you lose will never come back!

Keep on keeping on.
You can do it!

Make up your mind and go for it!
Give it everything you've got!
Do more than you've ever done.
Go the extra mile.
Beat the odds.
Take the first step.
Get going and don't stop.
Don't quit!
Keep your eyes on your goal.
Aim high.
Dream big.
See the possibilities.
Do what it takes to win.
You're gonna make it!
Stay focused.
Be persistent.
Make it happen!
It is possible.
There's no excuse for failure.
Face your fears.
Expect to win!
Believe in yourself!
Push yourself.
It's too soon to give up!
Get out of your comfort zone.
See it, say it, write it, have it!
It's never too late.
No one can stop you.
Just do it!
Try harder.
Never give up!
Go beyond what you have done.

Motivational Statements

Chapter One: *I can change my thoughts, my habits and my life. I can get and stay in the Life Cycle of Fitness and make health and fitness a way of life.*

Chapter Two: *I can change my thoughts to change my size, my habits and my lifestyle. Change is easy and I'm ready to change!*

Chapter Three: *I know exactly what to change and I expect to succeed.*

Chapter Four: *I can change my thoughts. I can change my life. I can lose weight. I can be successful.*

Chapter Five: *I can change. I can exercise. I love exercise. I can eat right. It's easy for me to give up foods that hinder my weight loss.*

Chapter Six: *I am good enough, smart enough and attractive enough!*

Chapter Seven: *I really want to change. I want to lose weight. I want to look and feel better. I want to eat right and exercise. I want to change more than I want to stay the same.*

Chapter Eight: *I can change, one step at a time. I keep my eyes on my goals, and I don't look back. I forget the past, it's a new day. I never give up because I have perserverance. To stay on track, I use my endurance.*

Chapter Nine: *It's easy for me to reach my goals when I take it one step at a time.*

Chapter Ten: *I have time for important things like exercise and eating right. There is time to stay healthy and lose weight.*

Chapter Eleven: *Planning my life is easy. Making new habits is easy.*

Chapter Twelve: *I love healthy foods. I love fresh fruits and vegetables. I can resist junk foods and candy. Sugar has no power over me.*

Chapter Thirteen: *I love exercise! It's fun and makes me feel great!*

Chapter Fourteen: *I eat when I'm hungry. I love natural foods. It's easy to know my natural body signals.*

Chapter Fifteen: *I know when I eat and I only eat when my body needs food.*

Chapter Sixteen: *I eat just what's right for me. It's easy to stop when I'm full.*

Chapter Seventeen: *It's easy to use a Food Diary. It helps me know what I'm eating.*

Order Form

Please Print

Name

Address

City   **State**   **Zip**

Phone

E-mail

METHOD OF PAYMENT:

Check   **Credit Card**   ☐ Visa   **OR**   ☐ Mastercard

Card #

Authorization Signature

ITEM	QTY	PRICE
Why Can't I Stay Motivated? ($14.95)		
Why Can't I Lose Weight? ($17.95)		
Why Can't I Lose Weight Cookbook ($17.95)		
Subtotal		
Shipping & Handling Add 15%		
Tax		
Total		

Please inquire about Lorrie's mini books and nutritional products.

Send check or money order to:

Life Design Nutrition
Lorrie Medford, CN
PO Box 54007
Tulsa, OK 74155
918-664-4483
E-mail orders: lorrie@lifedesignnutrition.com
www.lifedesignnutrition.com
Fax: 918-664-0300